THE COMPLETE COOKBOOK ON VEGAN CUISINE UPDATED 2021/22 FOR BEGINNERS

Vegan Cooking in all its nuances, a complete collection of all the most famous recipes that will allow you to balance your metabolism, will help you lose weight if you need it and you will immediately realize how much your body and your mind will benefit over time a healthy and natural lifestyle

Robert Verdini

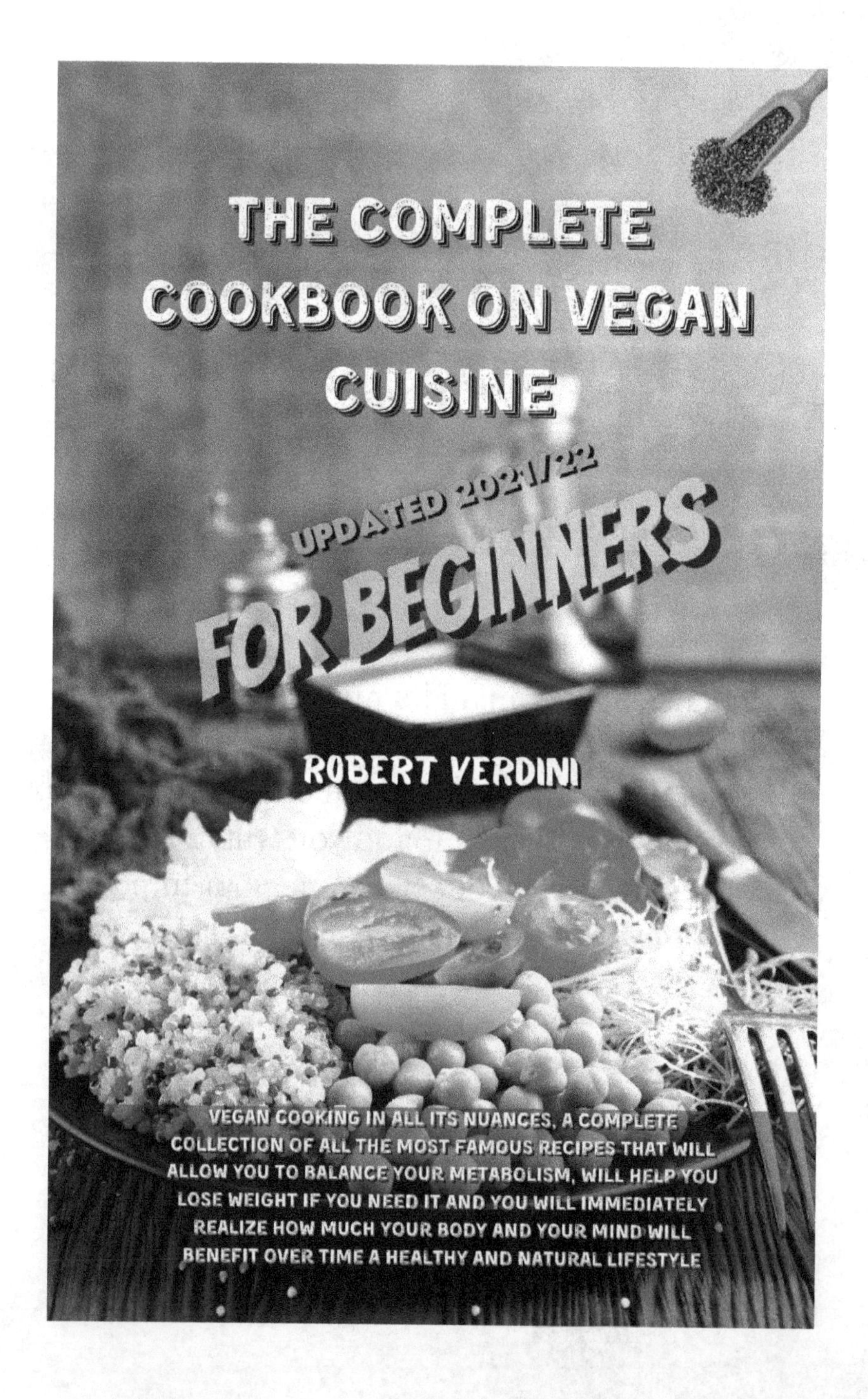
THE COMPLETE
COOKBOOK ON VEGAN
CUISINE
UPDATED 2021/22
FOR BEGINNERS
ROBERT VERDINI
VEGAN COOKING IN ALL ITS NUANCES, A COMPLETE
COLLECTION OF ALL THE MOST FAMOUS RECIPES THAT WILL
ALLOW YOU TO BALANCE YOUR METABOLISM, WILL HELP YOU
LOSE WEIGHT IF YOU NEED IT AND YOU WILL IMMEDIATELY
REALIZE HOW MUCH YOUR BODY AND YOUR MIND WILL
BENEFIT OVER TIME A HEALTHY AND NATURAL LIFESTYLE

Table Of Contents

The information in the following pages is broadly considered a truthful and accurate account of facts and as such, any inattention, use, or misuse of the information in question by the reader will render any resulting actions solely under their purview. There are no scenarios in which the publisher or the original author of this work can be in any fashion deemed liable for any hardship or damages that may befall them after undertaking information described herein.

Additionally, the information in the following pages is intended only for informational purposes and should thus be thought of as universal. As befitting its nature, it is presented without assurance regarding its prolonged validity or interim quality. Trademarks that are mentioned are done without written consent and can in no way be considered an endorsement from the trademark holder.

☆ *55% OFF for BookStore NOW at $ 30,95 instead of $ 41,95!* ☆

If you are a lover of Vegan cuisine or you are

about to learn more about it then this book is

for you, you will find many quick and easy

recipes to prepare from breakfast to dessert,

have fun and cook with love.

Buy is NOW and let your Customers get addicted to this amazing book!

Introduction

Veganism is a lifestyle that seeks to exclude, as far as possible and practicable, any form of exploitation and cruelty to animals, to get food, to make clothing or for any other reason.

The vegan diet is very different from the traditional diet; it includes all kinds of fruits, vegetables, nuts, cereals, seeds, beans and legumes, prepared according to many different recipes: from curry to desserts, from savory pies to pizza. However, it's not just about diet.

Vegans avoid exploiting animals for any reason, from making accessories to clothing, from using hygiene products to using elements of animal origin.

The alternatives found on the market today are now affordable. In this book there are many cheerful and tasty recipes, to prepare hearty breakfasts, delicious snacks, tasty sauces, colorful and unusual salads, tasty soups and inviting desserts, all made with vegan ingredients and much more...

Dive into the Vegan world and increase your cooking skills and surprise your friends and family.

BREAKFAST

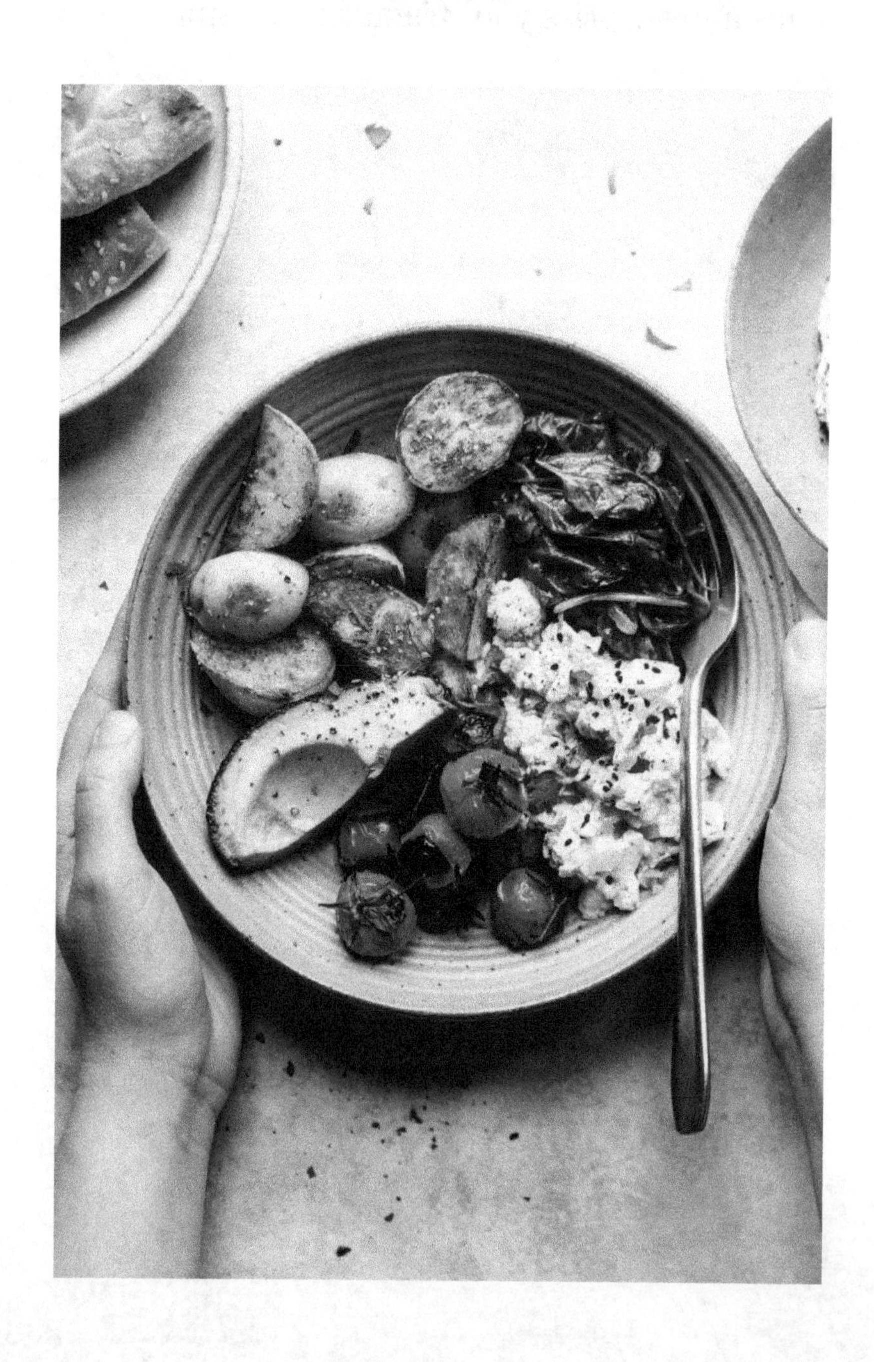

Breakfast Parfait

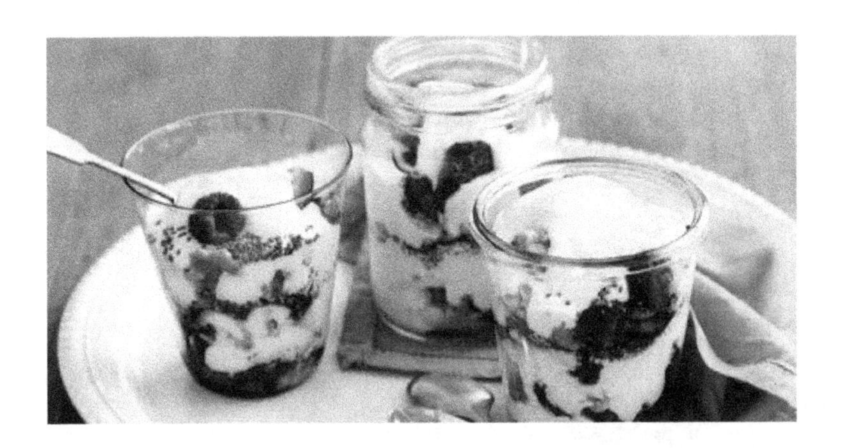

Servings:4
Ingredients:

24 oz. soy yogurt
1/4 cup maple syrup
2 cups cooked wheat berries
1/2 lb. fresh strawberries, sliced
6 oz. fresh blueberries
4 tsp. flax seeds

Directions:

Mix the yogurt and the maple syrup.
Arrange the ingredients in layers in 4 large glasses. First, put one-third of the yogurt in the glass base, followed by wheat berries, then top with the fruit.

Sprinkle 1 a teaspoon of the flax seeds over the top of each.

Oaty Apple Pancakes

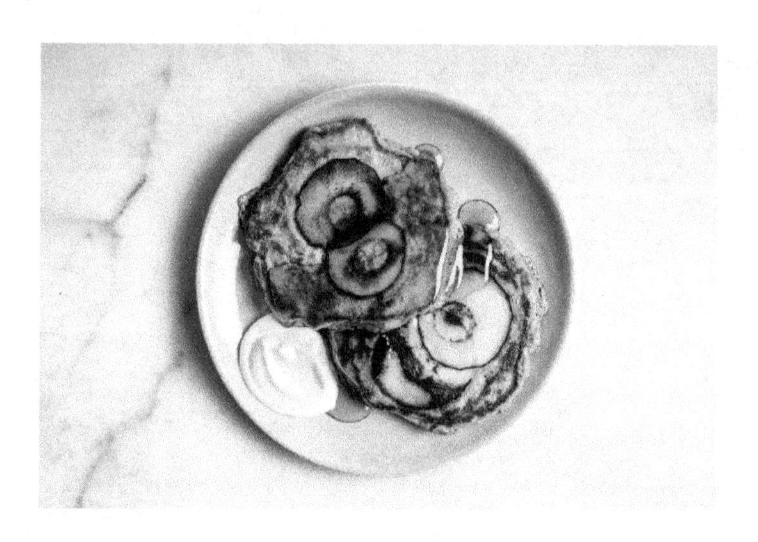

Servings:4
Ingredients:

1/2 cup all-purpose flour
1/2 cup quick-cooking oats
2 tsp. baking powder
1 tbsp. brown sugar
1 tbsp. vegetable oil
1 cup oat milk or apple juice
1 medium-tart apple, shredded
1 tsp. ground cinnamon
1–2 tbsp. sunflower oil, for frying,
warmed maple syrup, to serve

Directions:

Mix flour, oats, baking powder, sugar, vegetable oil, oat milk, shredded apple, and cinnamon together in a large mixing bowl.
Lightly oil a nonstick skillet or griddle with sunflower oil and place over medium heat.
Carefully pour about 1/4 cup of the pancake batter into the pan.
Fry on one side until lightly browned, then flip and cook the second side.
Keep warm. Repeat with the remaining batter. Serve with warmed maple syrup.
It makes 10–12 pancakes

Scrambled Tofu

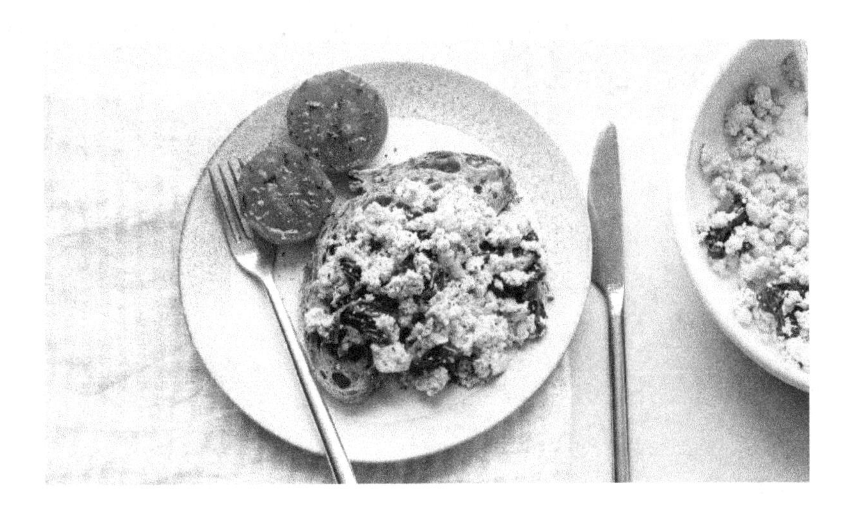

Servings:4
Ingredients:

1 (14-oz.) package firm tofu
1 tbsp. vegetable oil
1 small onion, chopped
1 clove garlic, minced
1 tsp. powdered turmeric
1–2 tbsp. soy sauce
black pepper

Directions:

Drain the crumble and tofu it with your hands into a plastic medium bowl.

Heat the oil in a skillet over medium heat and gently fry the onion and garlic until softened, 6/8 minutes. Add the powdered turmeric, then stir in the tofu. Reduce the heat slightly and season with soy sauce and black pepper to taste.
Serve hot.

French Toast

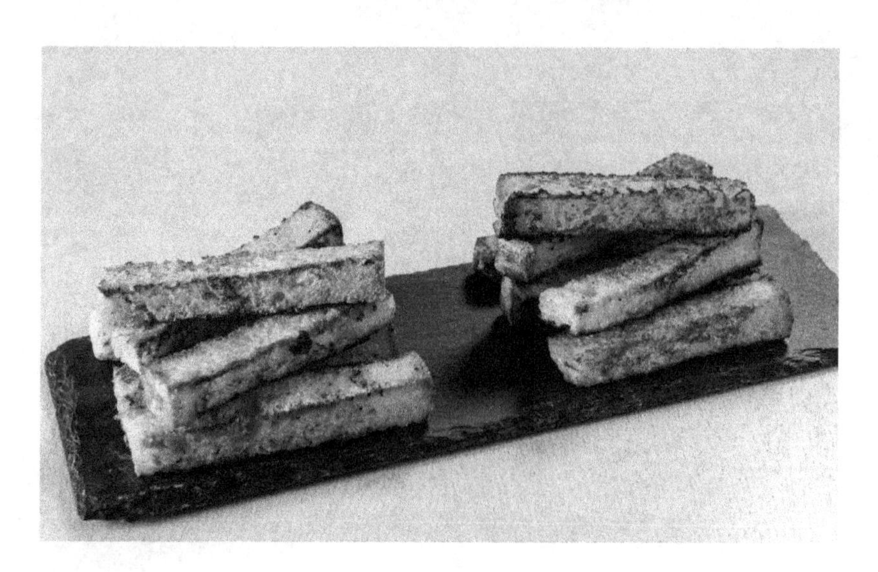

Servings:4
Ingredients:

2 tbsp. silken tofu
1 cup oat or soy milk
1 tbsp. nutritional yeast
1 tbsp. sugar
1 tsp. vanilla extract
1/2 tsp. ground cinnamon
pinch ground nutmeg
canola oil or non-dairy butter, for frying
8 slices bread
warmed maple syrup, to serve

Directions:

In a medium bowl, blend the tofu to a paste with a little of the oat or soy milk.
When smooth, add the remaining milk, nutritional yeast, sugar, vanilla, cinnamon, and nutmeg.
Lightly oil a large skillet or griddle with canola oil or non-dairy butter.
Dip the bread slices into the mixture, covering both sides. Cook over medium-low heat, flipping once, until golden on both sides. Cut into triangles and serve with warmed maple syrup.

Breakfast Bars

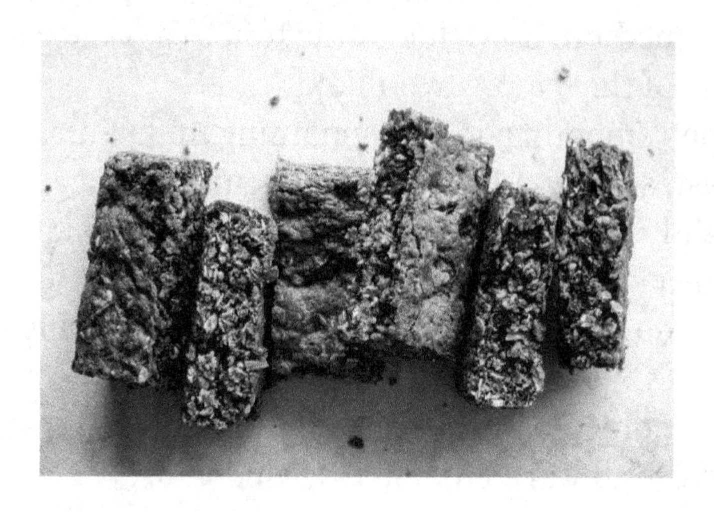

Servings:4
Ingredients:

1 cup quick-cooking rolled oats
1 cup whole wheat flour
1/2 cup brown sugar
1/4 tsp. baking soda
1/4 tsp. salt
1/4 tsp. ground cinnamon
pinch ground nutmeg
1/4 cup sunflower seeds
1/4 cup shredded coconut
1/4 cup dried cranberries
1 tbsp. flax seeds
1 tbsp. sesame seeds
1/2 cup canola oil

3 tbsp. cranberry juice

Directions:

Heat oven to 300°F and lightly oil an 9×9-inch baking pan.
Combine all the dry ingredients, then stir in the oil and cranberry juice and mix well.
Put the mixture into the baking pan 9 x9 and bake for 30–35 minutes until browned.
Let the loaf cool for 7 minutes, then cut into slices.
Store in an airtight container for 1 or 2 week or longer.

Fluffy Pancakes

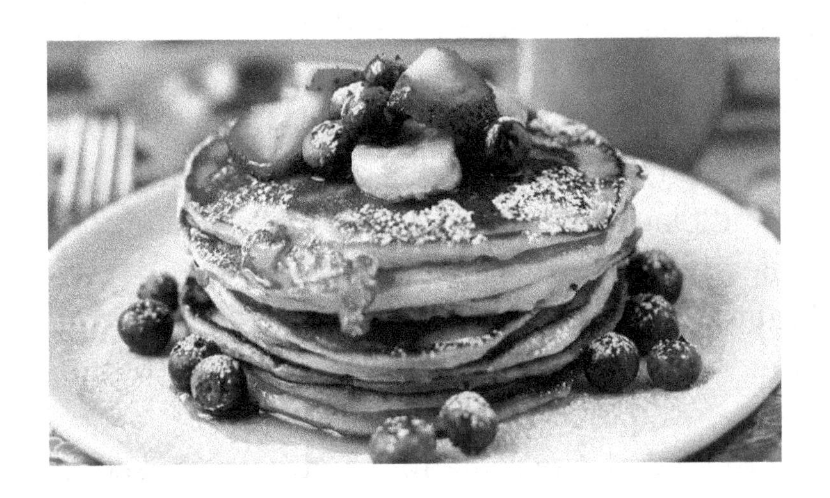

Servings:4
Ingredients:

2 cups all-purpose flour
1 heaping tbsp. soy flour
2 tsp. baking powder
1/2 tsp. baking soda
pinch salt
2 tbsp. sugar
2 cups plus 2 tbsp. soy milk
1/2 tsp. vanilla extract
sunflower oil, for frying,
warmed maple syrup and non-dairy butter, to serve

Directions:

In a large bowl, combine flour, soy flour, baking powder, baking soda, salt, and sugar. Add the vanilla,soy milk and stir until you have quite a thick batter.

Lightly oil a nonstick skillet or griddle with sunflower oil and place over medium heat. Gently pour a ladleful of batter into the pan.

Wait until bubbles appear all over the surface of the pancake, then flip it over and cook on the other side until golden brown.

Continue with the remaining batter while keeping the cooked pancakes warm under a clean cloth.

Stack the pancakes on small plates, and serve with warmed maple syrup and nondairy butter.

Orange Marmalade Bran Muffins

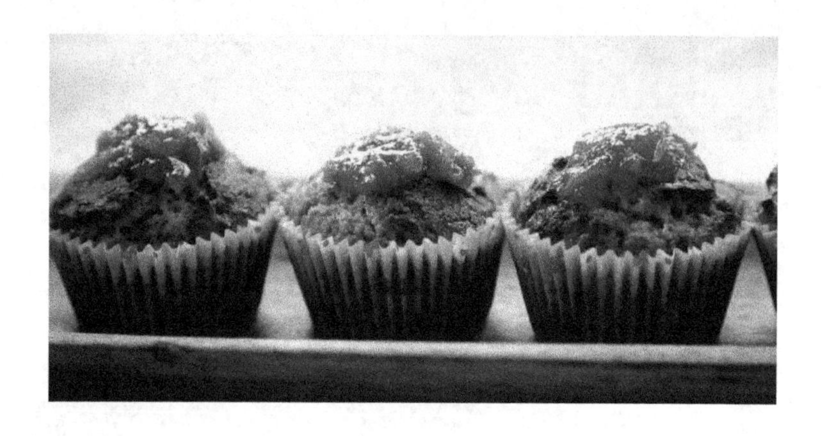

Servings:4
Ingredients:

1 1/2 cups wheat bran
1/2 cup boiling water
1/4 cup canola oil
3/4 cup brown sugar
egg replacer
1 cup soy milk
1 1/4 cups whole wheat flour
1 1/4 tsp. baking soda
1/2 tsp. salt
1 cup orange marmalade

Directions:

Line a muffin pan with paper cups.Preheat oven to 400°F.
In a plastic medium bowl, mix together all the ingredients.
Spoon into the muffin cups, filling to about the three-quarters level.
Bake the muffins for about 20 minutes until well risen and springy to the touch.
Cool for 5/8 minutes, then transfer the muffins to a wire rack to finish cooling.

VEGAN DISHES

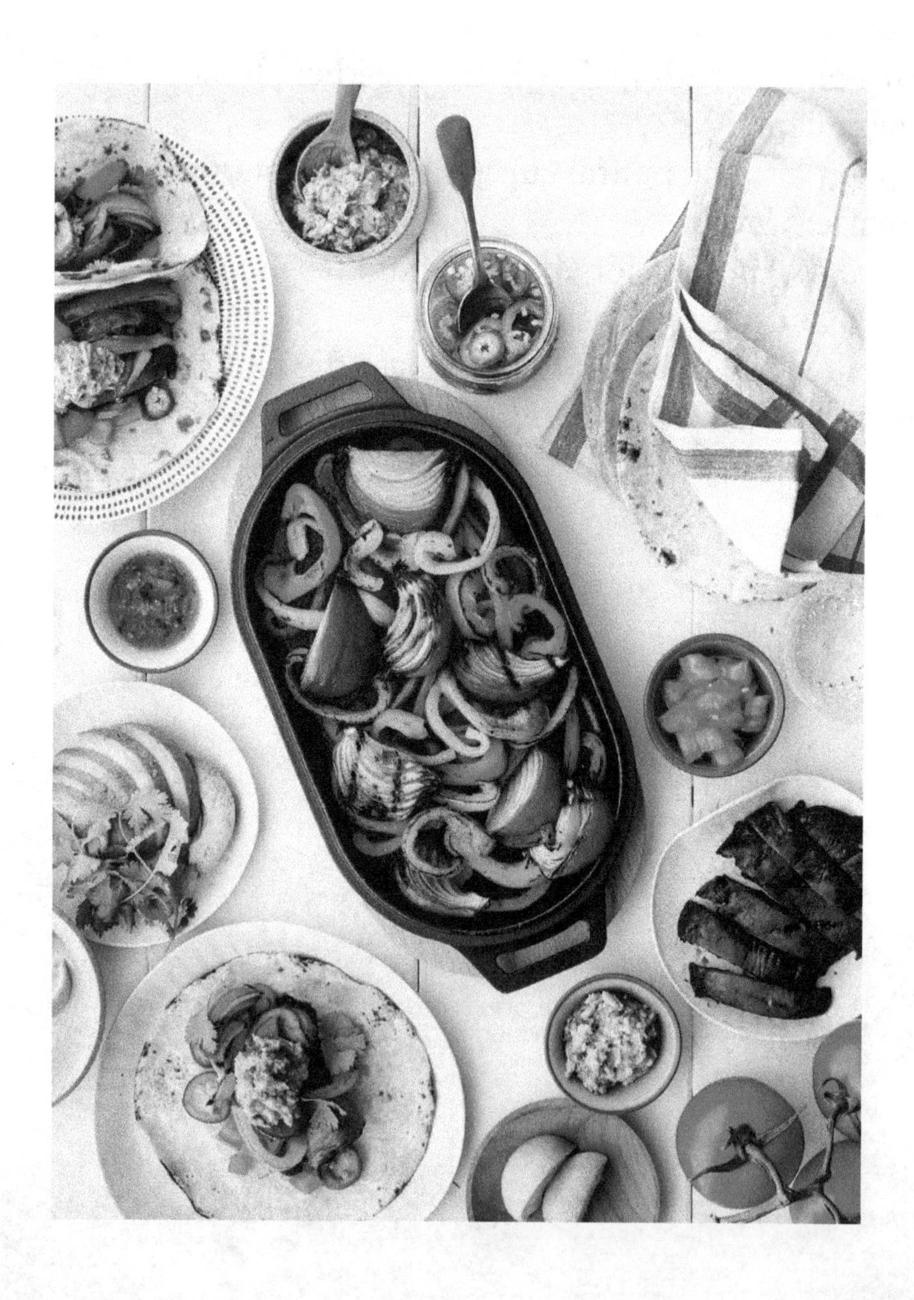

Bissara

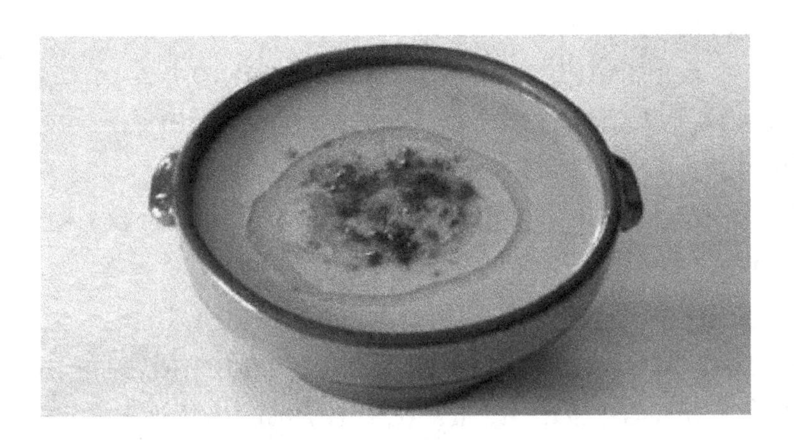

Servings:4
Ingredients:

2 cups large dried fava beans, soaked overnight and drained
3 cloves garlic
1/2 cup olive oil
8 cups water
1 small green chile, seeded and chopped
3 tbsp. lemon juice
1 tsp. ground cumin
sea salt and black pepper
paprika
chopped fresh parsley to garnish

Directions:

Place the fava beans, garlic, 1/4 cup olive oil, and water in a saucepan.
Bring to a boil, then cook over medium heat until the beans are tender, about 1 to the hour, depending on the size and freshness of the beans.
Drain and cool, reserving 1 1/2 cups of the cooking liquor.
Place the beans and the green chile in a food processor with 1 cup of the reserved liquor. Blend until smooth, adding more liquid if necessary to obtain a firmer puree.
Return the purée to a clean saucepan and stir in the lemon juice, cumin, and salt and pepper to taste.
Cook gently for 5 minutes, stirring.
Transfer the bissara to a serving bowl.
Drizzle with the remaining olive oil, sprinkle with paprika to taste, and garnish with parsley.
Serve at room temperature with flatbread and vegetable sticks, if desired.

Tomato Bruschetta

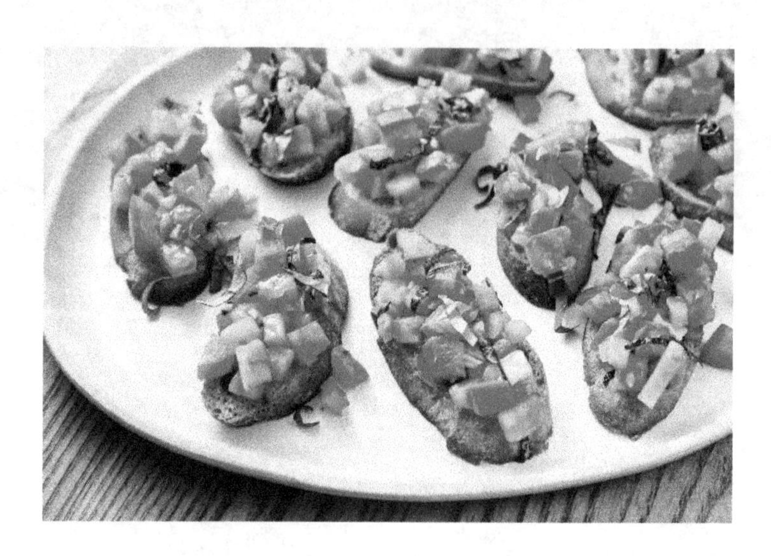

Servings:6
Ingredients:

4 large, thick slices ciabatta
1 garlic clove, halved
2 tbsp. extra-virgin olive oil
sea salt and black pepper
3 fresh tomatoes, skinned, seeded, and chopped
8 sun-dried tomatoes in oil, roughly chopped
1/2 cup torn fresh basil leaves
oil from jar of sun-dried tomatoes

Directions:

Rub each slice of ciabatta with the garlic clove.
Preheat the oven to 375°F.
Put all the bread on a baking sheet and drizzle with the olive oil. Season with salt and bake for about 10 minutes, turning once, until golden.
Mix the tomatoes, sun-dried tomatoes, and half the basil together.
Season to taste with salt and pepper.
Place on top of the ciabatta slices and arrange on a baking sheet.
Drizzle with a little of the oil from the sun-dried tomatoes. Return to the oven for 5 minutes to heat through.
Serve garnished with the rest of the basil.

Saffron Rice

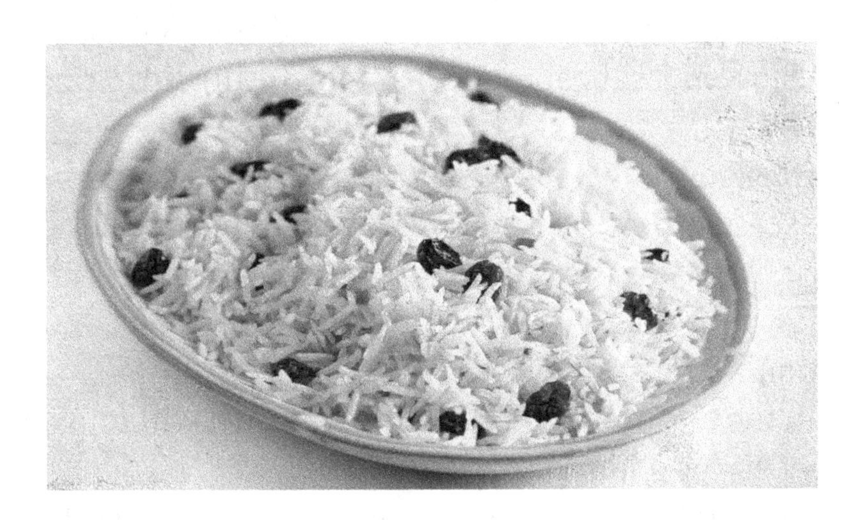

Servings:6
Ingredients:

3 1/2 cups vegetable bouillon
1/2 tsp. Saffron threads, soaked in 1 tbsp. hot water
2 bay leaves
1 (2-inch) cinnamon stick
2 whole cloves
1/2 tsp. sea salt
1/2 tsp. dried chili flakes (optional)
2 cups Thai jasmine rice or white basmati rice
1 tsp. lemon juice

Directions:

Put the bouillon, saffron and soaking water, bay leaves, cinnamon, cloves, salt, and chili flakes, if using, in a saucepan with a tight-fitting lid. Bring to a boil.

If using basmati rice, wash thoroughly to remove excess starch; jasmine rice does not need prewashing.

Add the rice to the pan, stir, cover, and simmer over low heat for 10–15 min, until the rice is cook and the liquid is absorbed.

Remove from the heat and, keeping the lid in place, let sit for 5 minutes.

Discard the bay leaves and cinnamon stick, add the lemon juice, taste, and adjust the seasoning. Fluff with a fork before serving.

Appams

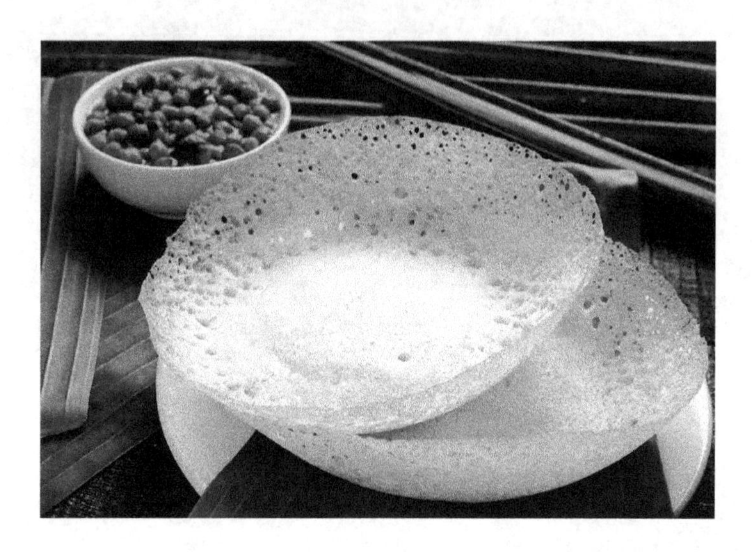

Servings:6
Ingredients:

2 tbsp. semolina
2 2/3 cups water
2 cups rice flour
1 tsp. sugar
1 tsp. rapid-rise yeast
1/2 cup full-fat coconut milk
1 tsp. sea salt

Directions:

Put the semolina and 2 cups water in a pan over moderate heat.
Bring to a boil, stirring continuously, then reduce the heat to low.
Cook and stir until a smooth paste is formed; transfer to a bowl and let cool. Add the rice flour, sugar, and yeast. Stir in the coconut milk and remaining water to form a thick batter.
Cover with plastic wrap and let rise in a warm place for 3–4 hours, until the batter is bubbly and doubled in volume.
Very carefully stir in the salt without beating the ai out of the mixture.
Heat an oiled griddle or nonstick skillet over a moderately high heat until very hot, add a ladleful of batter, and spread it out by swirling the pan to form a thin pancake.
Cover and cook for 3–4 minutes on one side only so that the base is lightly browned but the top remains very slightly moist; remove from the pan, keep warm and repeat with the remaining mixture.

Caramelized Onion

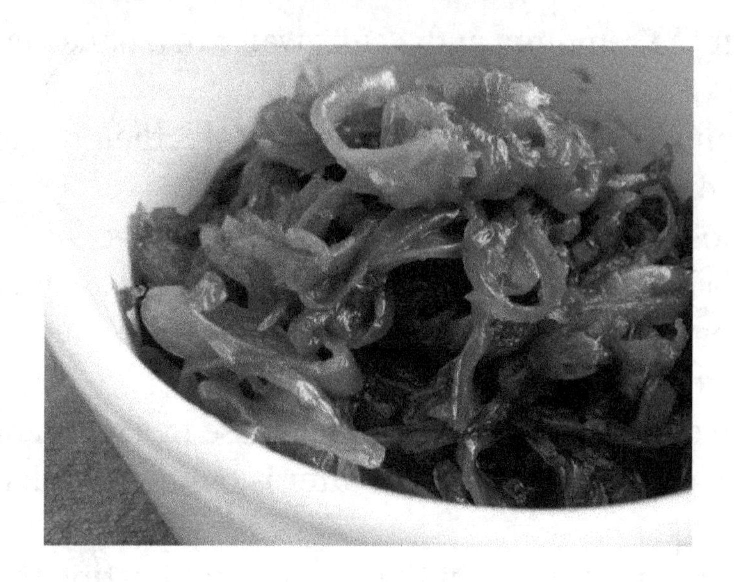

Servings:6
Ingredients:

2 tbsp. soy margarine
24 baby onions or shallots
Four small sprigs of fresh thyme
2 tbsp. balsamic vinegar
2 tsp. sugar
sea salt and black pepper
4 (12-inch) square pieces of parchment paper

Directions:

Preheat oven to 400°F.

Melt the margarine in a pan and add the onions, shaking well to coat the onions evenly in margarine. Put one-quarter of the onions and a sprig of thyme in the center of each of the paper squares, drizzle 1/2 tablespoon balsamic vinegar over each, then sprinkle with sugar, salt, and pepper.
Fold up the squares.
It doesn't matter how you do this, but make sure that the seams are well rolled — the packets expand with steam during cooking so they need to be well sealed.
Place on a cookie sheet in the oven and cook for 15 minutes, then shake the packets gently to move the contents about slightly, and cook for another 30 minutes, until the onions feel soft if carefully squeezed through a cloth.

Creamed Spinach

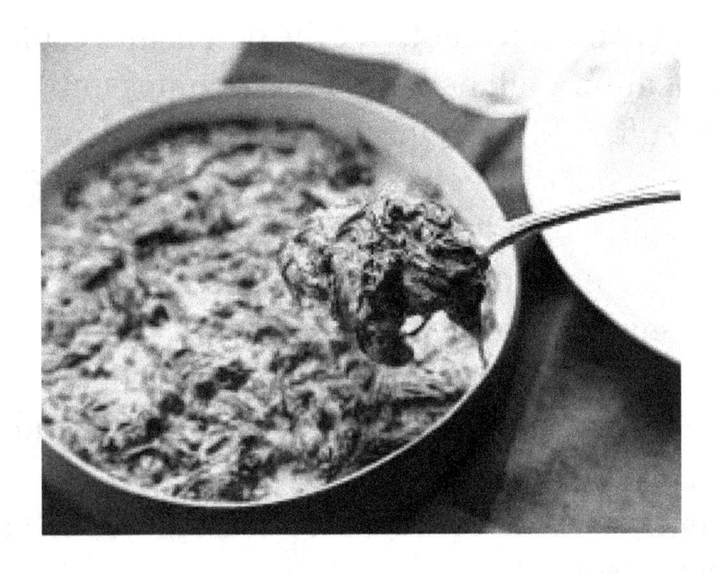

Servings:6
Ingredients:

1 tbsp. olive oil
1 small onion, finely chopped
1 garlic clove, minced
1 lb. fresh baby spinach, washed
1 cup non-dairy cream cheese
1/2 cup nondairy mayonnaise
1/4 cup nutritional yeast
1/4 tsp. garlic granules
1/4 tsp. ground nutmeg
sea salt and black pepper
3 tbsp. toasted slivered almonds to garnish

Directions:

Heat the olive oil in a pot, put the onion, and cook over a medium-high heat for a few minutes until the onion is soft. Add the minced garlic and cook another minute.
Add the spinach and cook with only the water clinging to the washed leaves until just tender; drain and transfer to a warmed serving dish.
Meanwhile, combine the nondairy cream cheese, mayonnaise,nutritional yeast, garlic granules, and nutmeg in a saucepan.
Heat gently without boiling, then season with salt and pepper to taste.
Pour the sauce over the spinach, toss gently, and garnish with the toasted almonds.

Triple Tomato Risotto

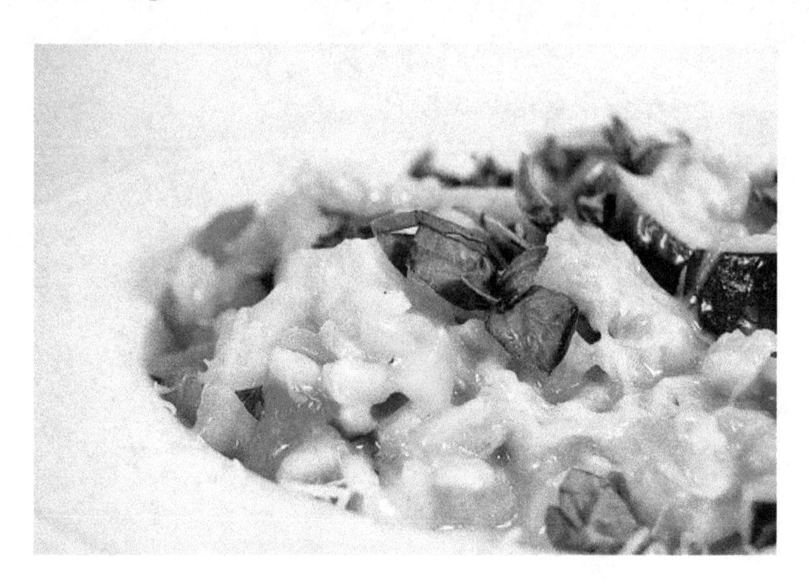

Servings:6
Ingredients:

12 oz. cherry tomatoes halved
8 garlic cloves, unpeeled
1 tbsp. olive oil
4 cups good vegetable bouillon
1 (15-oz.) can tomato sauce
1 tbsp. oil from sun-dried tomatoes
1 tbsp. soy margarine
4 shallots, finely chopped
2 cups arborio (risotto) rice
1/2 cup white wine
1/4 cup sun-dried tomatoes, finely chopped
1/2 cup chopped fresh basil

sea salt and black pepper

Directions:

Preheat oven to 400°F. Put the cherry tomatoes and the unpeeled garlic in a single layer in an oiled baking dish and drizzle with the olive oil.
Bake for about 25/30 minutes until the tomatoes have shriveled. Cool slightly, squeeze the flesh out of the garlic, mash with a fork, and set aside. In a medium pan, heat the bouillon and the tomato sauce until very hot; keep hot. Heat the tomato oil and margarine in a saucepan on medium-high heat, then add the shallots and cook for 5–7 minutes until the shallots are soft. Add the rice and stir to coat it with oil, then cook until the grains become translucent, about 2 minute. Add the wine and cook, stirring until absorbed, then add about one ladleful of the hot bouillon mixture and continue to cook, frequently stirring, until fully absorbed.
Add another ladleful of bouillon and allow it to be absorbed before adding another.
Continue this process until the rice is tender but still firm and just coated in a thick creamy sauce, about 20 minutes (you may not need all the bouillon). Very gently stir in the roasted cherry tomatoes, mashed garlic, sun-dried tomatoes, and basil, and season with salt and pepper to taste. Serve immediately.

Sicilian Caponata

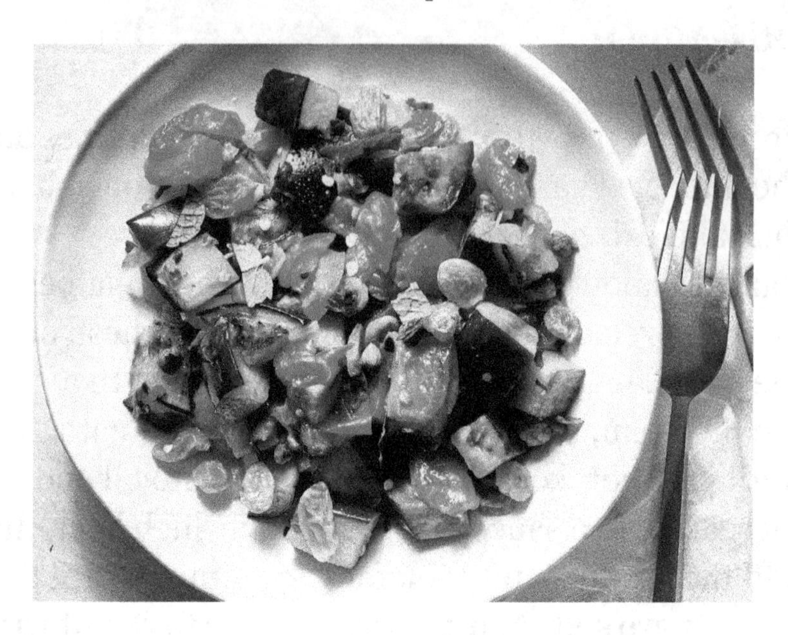

Servings:6
Ingredients:

2 large purple eggplants
sea salt
2 tbsp. salted capers
2–3 tbsp. olive oil
1 small red onion, finely chopped
2 stalks celery, chopped
2 garlic cloves, minced
1 tsp. dried oregano
2 tbsp. balsamic vinegar
2 tbsp. chopped fresh flat-leaf parsley

6 fresh tomatoes, skinned and chopped, or 1 (15-oz. can) chopped tomatoes
8 pitted green olives, halved
black pepper
1 tsp. sugar
8 oz. spaghetti
olive oil, to toss

Directions:

Cut the eggplant into 1-inch-thick slices, then sprinkle with salt. Leave for 1 hour, then wipe away the bitter juices with a paper towel.
Cut into large chunks. Meanwhile, put the capers in water to soak; drain.
Heat 2 tablespoons olive oil in a skillet and fry the eggplant slices in batches over medium-high heat, frequently stirring until they are just golden all over but not cooked through.
Add a little more oil, if required, and do not overcook.
Stir in the onion, celery, garlic, and oregano.
Continue to cook for about 5 minutes until the onion is soft and transparent.
Pour in the vinegar and cook, stirring, until it has evaporated, then add the capers, parsley, tomatoes, and olives.
Season to taste with salt, pepper, and sugar; cover, and cook for 15–20 minutes until the eggplant is tender.

Meanwhile, cook the spaghetti following the package directions until al dente. Drain, toss with a little olive oil, and serve immediately with the eggplant sauce.

Pasta with green Beans & Tomatoes

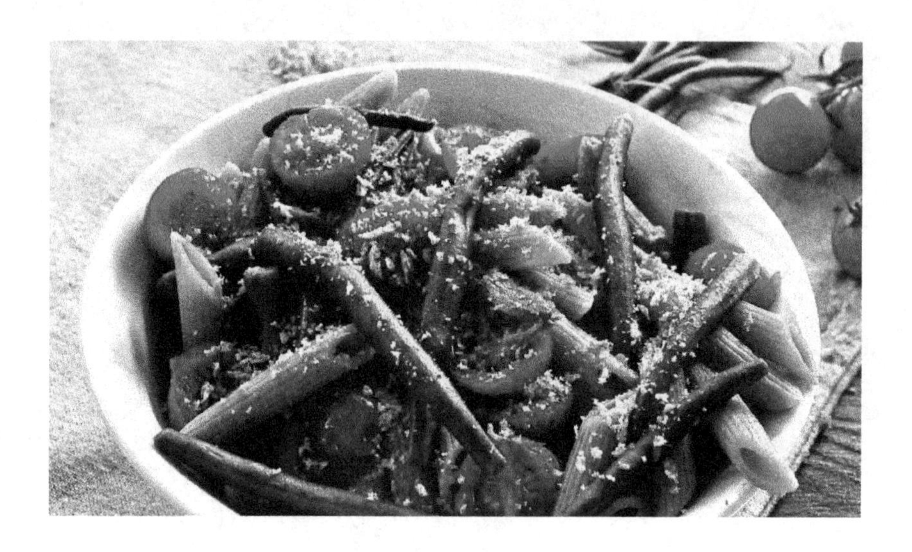

Servings:6
Ingredients:

2 tbsp. olive oil
1 medium onion, chopped
3 garlic cloves, crushed
1 (2-lb.) can crushed tomatoes
2 tbsp. sun-dried tomato paste
1/2 cup vegetable bouillon
2/3 cup red wine plus 1 tbsp. nutritional yeast
1 lb. fresh green beans
2 tsp. dried Italian herbs
1/2 tsp. sugar

sea salt and black pepper
1 lb. fusilli or pasta
olive oil, to coat
fresh basil, to garnish

Directions:

Heat the oil in a skillet, add the onion, then cook over a medium-high heat for 5–7 minutes or until the onion is soft, then add the crushed garlic.
Add the tomatoes, tomato paste, bouillon, wine, green beans, herbs, and sugar.
Season with salt and pepper. Bring to a boil, then cook for 20–25 minutes until the green beans are tender.
Cook the pasta in boiling water for about 10 minutes, or according to the package directions.
The pasta should be cooked through but still firm.
Drain, toss with olive oil, and serve coated with the sauce and garnished with basil.

Squash & Apricot Tagine

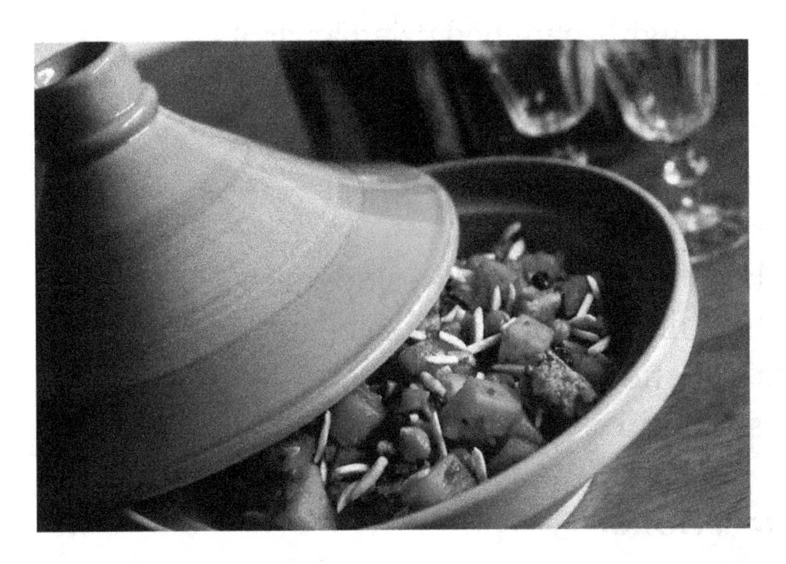

Servings:4
Ingredients:

1 small zucchini, roughly chopped
1/4 cup olive oil
1 onion, finely chopped
2 cloves garlic, minced
1-inch-piece gingerroot, finely shredded
1/2 tsp. ground cumin
1/2 tsp. ground turmeric
1 tsp. paprika
1/2 tsp. cayenne pepper
1 tsp. ground cinnamon
1 medium-large butternut squash, cut into chunks
2 medium potatoes, cut into chunks

2 carrots, thickly sliced
4 oz. green beans, sliced
1 cup roughly chopped dried apricots
1 1/2 cups vegetable bouillon
2 tsp. tomato paste
1 (15-oz.) can garbanzo beans
2 tsp. grated lemon zest
2 tbsp. finely chopped fresh parsley
2 tbsp. finely chopped fresh cilantro
sea salt and black pepper
fresh cilantro, to garnish

Directions:

Place the zucchini in a pan of boiling water, simmer for 10 minutes, until very soft, drain, and cool. Blend to a smooth purée and set aside.
Meanwhile, heat the olive oil in a saucepan, add the onion, and cook over medium-high heat for 5–7 minutes until soft.
Add the ginger, the garlic and then add the cumin, turmeric, paprika, cayenne, and cinnamon and cook for 1 minute. Stir in the squash, potato, carrots, green beans, and apricots until they are coated in the spices. Add the bouillon and tomato paste and bring to a boil.
Cover, reduce the heat and simmer until the squash is tender about 20 minutes.

Add the garbanzo beans, lemon zest, parsley, cilantro, and the zucchini purée.
Season to taste with salt and pepper,and serve.

Fennel, bell pepper & tomato tart

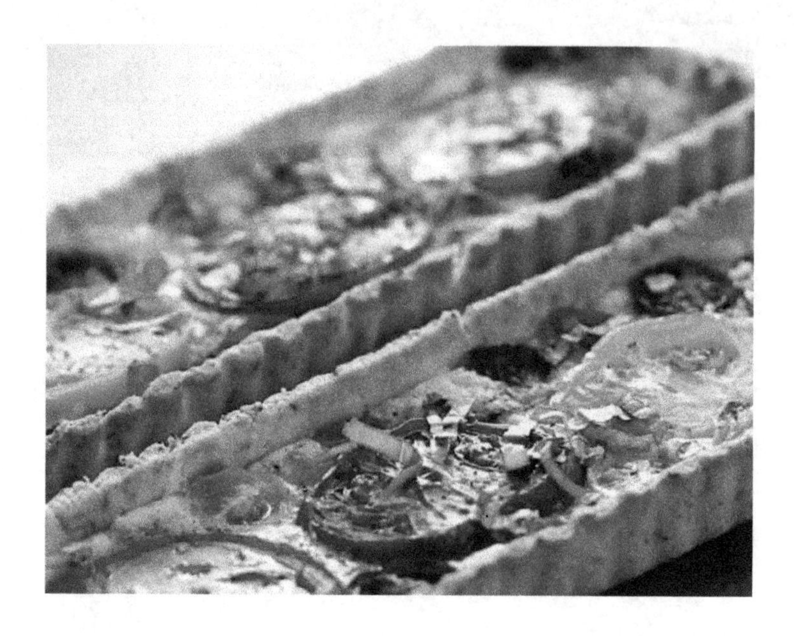

Servings:4
Ingredients:

1 (15-oz.) can navy beans
2 tbsp. nondairy milk
2 tbsp. vegan pesto
sea salt and pepper
2 heads fresh fennel
1 red bell pepper, seeded and halved
6 tomatoes, peeled and thickly sliced
1/2 tsp. coriander seeds

1/4 tsp. fennel seeds
2 1/2 tbsp. olive oil
1 tsp. lemon juice
1 sheet puff pastry

Directions:

Preheat oven to 375°F. In a food processor, combine the beans, nondairy milk, and pesto, and process until smooth. Season, and set aside.
Setup the base of the fennel, and remove and discard the long green stalks. Cut into 8 wedges and place in a saucepan. Cover with boiling water and simmer for 8 minutes, drain thoroughly, and cool. Meanwhile, put the bell pepper under a hot broiler and cook until the skin blackens, turn and repeat until the whole pepper is charred. Wrap in plastic wrap, let cool, then remove the skin and slice. Carefully unwrap the pastry and lay it on parchment paper on a cookie sheet. (If you can't find pastry sheets, roll out the pastry into a rectangle 1/8 inch thick.) With a sharp knife, score a border 1 inch from the edge – this will rise to form the edge of the tart. Spread the bean purée on top of the pastry, taking care to stay within the scored line. Put the tomato slices on top, followed by the fennel and pepper.
Lightly crush the coriander and fennel seeds and sprinkle over the vegetables with a little salt and pepper. Brush the outside border with olive oil, then

drizzle the remaining oil and lemon juice over the vegetables.

Bake for about 20 minutes, or until the pastry is risen and golden brown. Slip off the parchment paper and serve warm.

Pumpkin & Tofu Kebabs

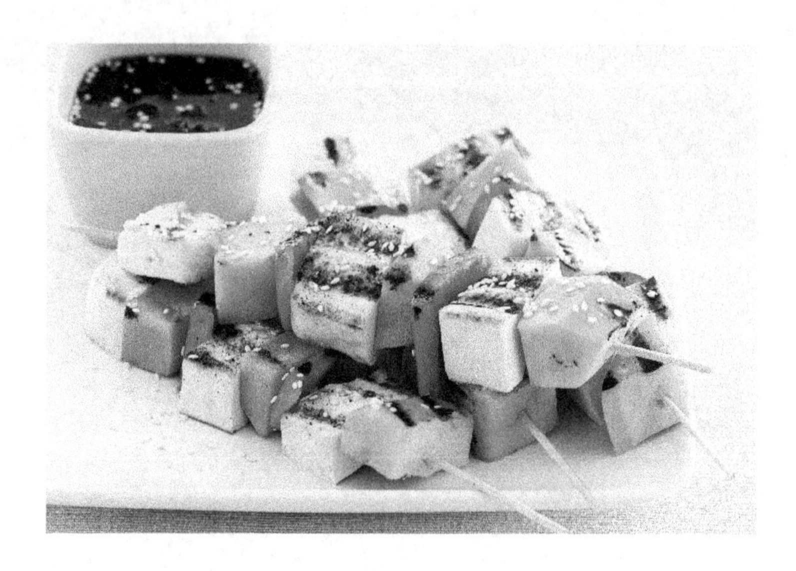

Servings:4
Ingredients:

8 baby potatoes
1 (12-oz.) young pumpkin
1 large zucchini
2 red, green, peppers, seeded
2 small red onions
8 cherry tomatoes
12 oz. smoked firm tofu, cut into 1-inch cubes
oil, to brush
for the glaze
1/2 cup olive oil
1 1/2 tbsp. cider or white wine vinegar

2 tbsp. maple syrup
2 tbsp. orange juice
2 tbsp. chopped fresh parsley
1 tbsp. chopped fresh rosemary
2 tbsp. Dijon mustard

Directions:

Cook the baby potatoes in a small pan of boiling water until almost cooked; drain and pat dry.
Meanwhile, mix the ingredients for the frosting.
Cut the pumpkin, zucchini, and bell pepper into 1-inch pieces. Cut the onions into quarters.
Put the potatoes and vegetables in a shallow dish or container.
Pour marinade over vegetables. Cover and refrigerate for at least about 2 hours.
Heat the grill to medium and brush with a little oil.
Alternately thread the vegetables and tofu onto 8 skewers, leaving a little space between each.
Put the skewers on the grill and cook, turning frequently and basting with the marinade for about 10 minutes. Remove when the pumpkin and zucchini are tender-crisp.

Winter Vegetable Bake

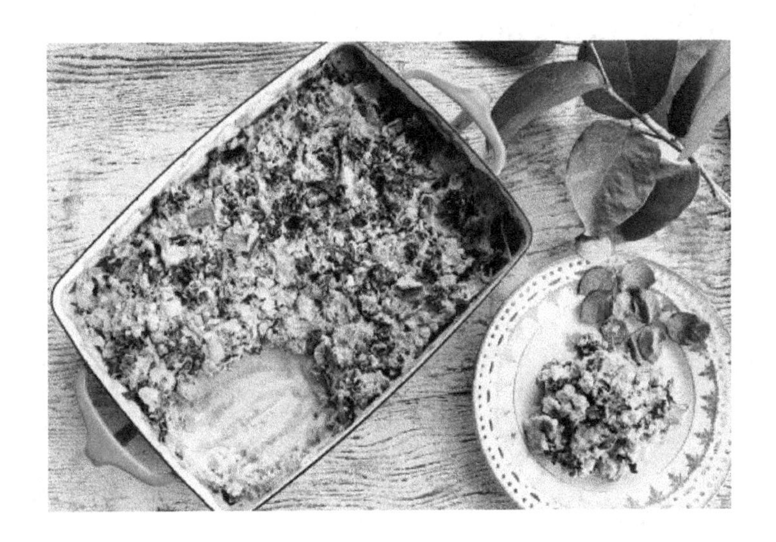

Servings:4
Ingredients:

2 tbsp. olive oil
2 red onions, cut into wedges
1/2 butternut squash, diced
1/2 rutabaga, diced
3 medium carrots, thickly sliced
2 medium leeks, trimmed and sliced
2 medium parsnips, thickly sliced
3 raw beets, quartered
2 celery stalks, sliced
1 tsp. caraway seeds
2 garlic cloves, minced

3 tbsp. tomato paste
1 1/4 cups vegetable bouillon
1 (14-oz.) can crushed tomatoes
1 tsp. mixed dried herbs
sea salt and pepper
1 tbsp. cornstarch
1 tbsp. water
for the biscuits
2 cups flour
1 tbsp. baking powder
1/2 tsp. salt
1 tsp. dried rosemary
4 tbsp. soy margarine
3/4 cup soy milk
soy milk, to glaze

Directions:

Heat the oil in a heavy-duty, ovenproof skillet, then add the onions, squash, rutabagas, carrots, leeks, parsnips, beet, celery, caraway seeds, and garlic. Cooking over high heat for 5 minutes or until the onions are soft.
Add the tomato paste, bouillon, crushed tomatoes, and their juices and herbs. Season to taste. Bring to a boil for 30 minutes, cover.
Stir the cornstarch into the water, add a little of the pan juices, then pour the mixture into the pan, stirring, until the liquid thickens a little. Meanwhile,

to make the biscuits, put all the dry ingredients into a bowl. Blend in the margarine with your fingertips or a fork until the mixture resembles fine breadcrumbs. Add the soy milk and stir until a soft, smooth dough is formed, adding more flour if the dough is sticky. Roll out the dough 3/4 inch thick on a lightly floured surface and stamp out 8 to 9 rounds with a 2-inch cookie cutter.

Preheat oven to 400°F.

Arrange biscuits around the edge of the vegetable mixture, brush the tops with soy milk, and bake for 20 minutes, or until risen and golden brown.

Pepperoncini & Tofu Sandwiches

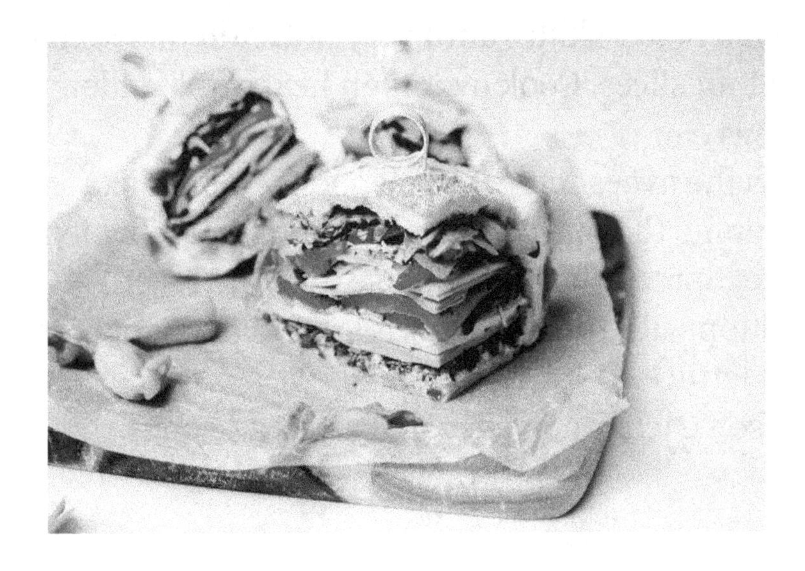

Servings:2
Ingredients:

1 tsp. sunflower oil
6 oz. firm tofu
1/2 ripe avocado, sliced
1 1/2 tsp. lemon juice
4 tbsp. nondairy mayonnaise
4 slices whole-wheat sandwich bread
2 large tomato
3 small peperoncini peppers, stems removed and sliced lengthwise

lettuce leaves
sea salt and black pepper

Directions:

Heat a heavy skillet until very hot. Add the oil, then the tofu slices. Cook over high heat until golden brown.
Toss the avocado in 1/2 teaspoon lemon juice.
Combine the mayonnaise with the remaining lemon juice. Spread the mayonnaise over the bread, and top with the tofu, avocado, tomato, pepperoncini, and lettuce.
Season each sandwich with salt and pepper.

Mixed Vegetable Stir-Fry

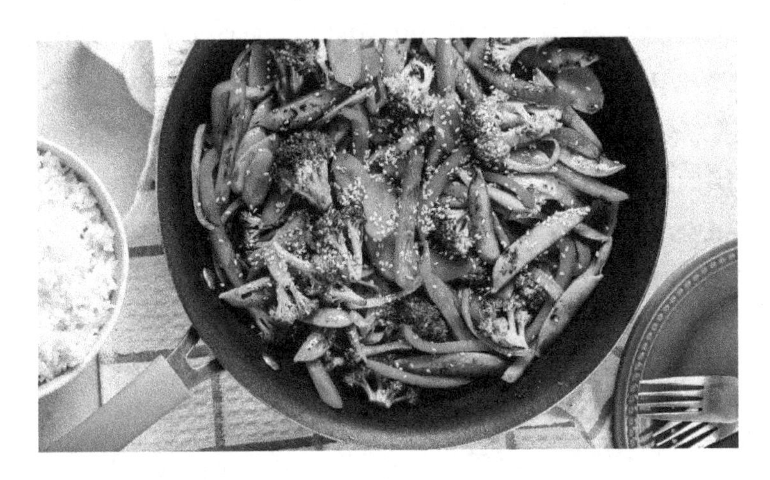

Servings:2
Ingredients:

8 oz. rice or wheat noodles
1 tbsp. peanut or vegetable oil
1 red chile pepper, sliced
1 garlic clove, sliced
1 lb. mixed fresh vegetables such as bok choy, snow peas, baby corn, and broccoli florets
2 tbsp. soy sauce
2 1/2 tbsp. sweet chili sauce
2 cups bean sprouts
2 tsp. sesame oil

Directions:

Cook the noodles for few minutes; drain.

Heat the oil in a large pan, and fry the chile and garlic for 1 minute.
Add the mixed vegetables and stir-fry over a high heat for 3 minutes. Add the soy sauce and chili sauce, and toss to coat.
Put the bean sprouts and continue to stir-fry for 2–3 minutes until the vegetables are tender-crisp. Toss with the noodles and drizzle with the sesame oil; serve immediately.

Black Bean Soup

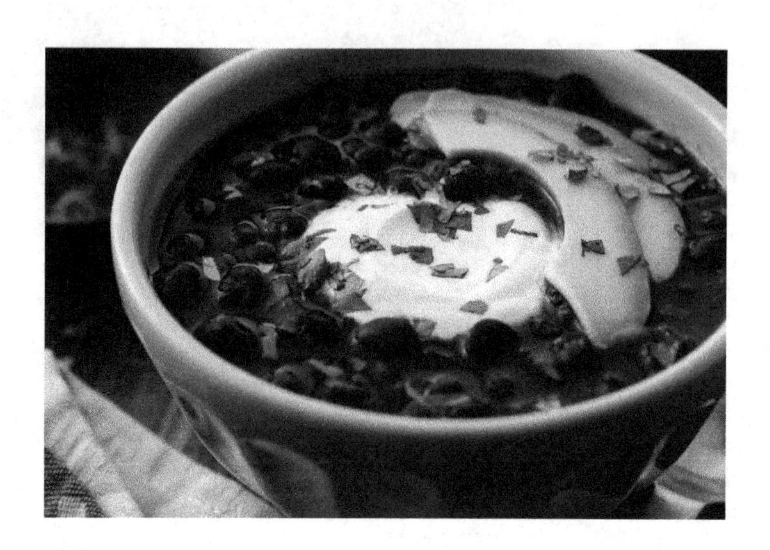

Servings:2
Ingredients:

2 cups black beans, soaked in cold water overnight or at least 5 hours (or 3 15-oz. cans black beans)
1/3 cup olive oil
2 medium white onions, finely chopped
3 garlic cloves, minced
1 carrot, chopped
1–2 fresh red chiles, chopped
2 tsp. ground cumin
1/4 tsp. smoked paprika
2 bay leaves
4 cups vegetable bouillon

1 (14.5-oz.) can whole or chopped tomatoes
small bunch of fresh thyme, stalks removed

for garnish
1 small red onion, sliced
chopped fresh cilantro
juice of 1 lime

Directions:

For dried beans only, drain the beans and put them in a saucepan with 5 cups of water over a high heat. Bring to a boil and boil rapidly for 10 minutes, then reduce heat and simmer for 1 1/4 to 1 1/2 hours until soft. Drain. Heat the oil in a skillet, then add the onion and cook over medium-high heat for 5 minutes when the onion is soft. Add the minced garlic, carrot, chiles, cumin, paprika, and bay leaves. Continue to cook for another 2 minutes. Add the beans with the bouillon, tomatoes, and thyme leaves. Bring to a boil, reduce the heat, cover, and simmer for 20 minutes. Remove the bay leaves, then take out 2 cups of the soup and blend with an immersion blender or in a food processor. Return the puréed soup to the pan, stir, and heat through. Season to taste with salt and pepper. Serve garnished with thin slices of red onion, chopped cilantro, and a squeeze of lime juice.

Minestrone

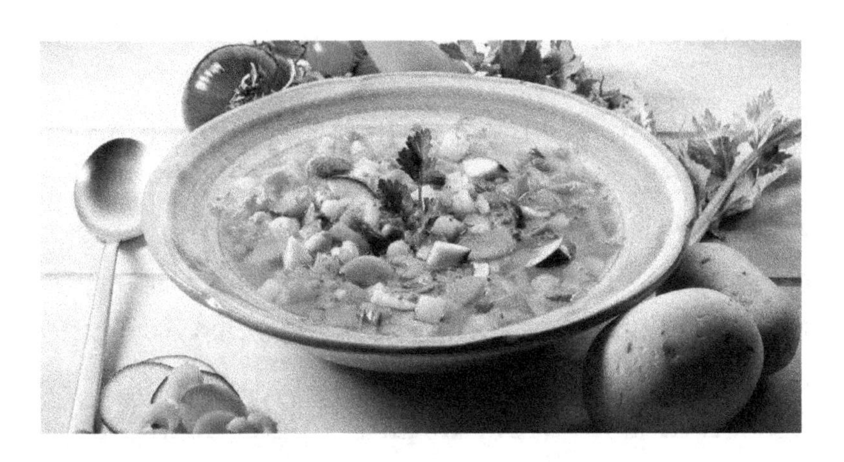

Servings:4
Ingredients:

1/2 cup olive oil
2 medium onions, chopped
2 carrots, chopped
2 stalks celery, sliced
1 cup sliced green beans
3 medium zucchini, chopped
3 cups shredded cabbage
8 cups vegetable bouillon
1 cup chopped canned tomatoes
2 tbsp. nutritional yeast
1 tsp. dried oregano
1/2 tsp. dried basil
sea salt and black pepper
1 (15-oz.) can white beans

1 cup orzo or other tiny pasta

Directions:

Heat oil in a very large skillet, then add onions and cook, stirring frequently for about 8 minutes until golden. Stir in each of the other vegetables in turn, cooking each one for 3 minutes before adding the next. Add the bouillon, tomatoes, yeast, oregano, and basil.
Season to taste with salt and pepper. Bring to a boil, then reduce the heat to very low, cover, and simmer for 2 hours. If making in advance, chill.
Reheat if required.
Add the beans and orzo and cook for 15 minutes before serving.

Corn & Jalapeño Chowder

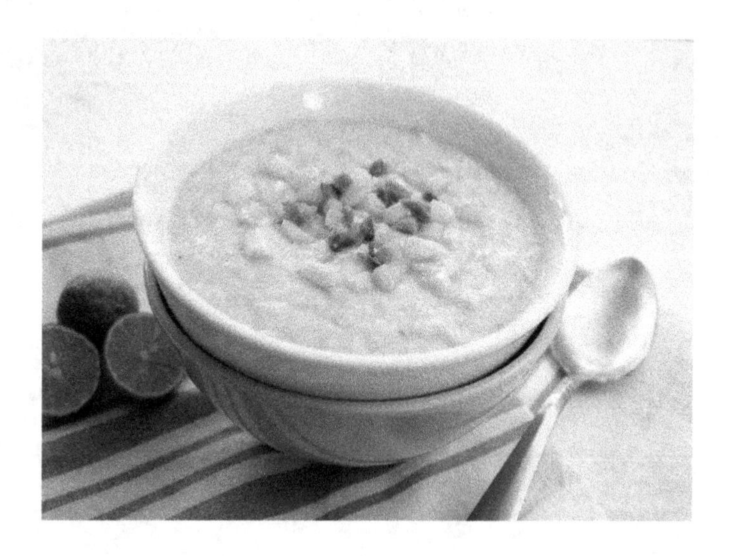

Servings:4
Ingredients:

4 large corn cobs, shucked and silks discarded (or 4 cups frozen corn)
2 tbsp. sunflower oil
1 large white onion, chopped
2 medium potatoes, chopped
1–2 jalapeño chiles, chopped
2 cups soy milk
1 vegetarian bouillon cube
sea salt and black pepper
chopped fresh parsley to garnish

Directions:

If using fresh corn, put the corn cobs in a large saucepan in boiling water and simmer for 10–12 minutes until tender. Cool, reserving the cooking liquor. With a knife, remove the corn kernels.
Heat the oil in a large skillet, then add the onion and cook for 5–7 minutes over medium-high heat until soft.
Stir in the potatoes and the jalapeño to taste, and cook for 3 minutes more. Add 1 3/4 cups of strained reserved corn cooking liquor or water, the soy milk, bouillon, and corn.
Season to taste with salt and pepper.
Bring to a boil, then reduce the heat and simmer for about 10 minutes, or until the potatoes are tender but still retaining their shape. Serve garnished with chopped parsley.

Miso Soup

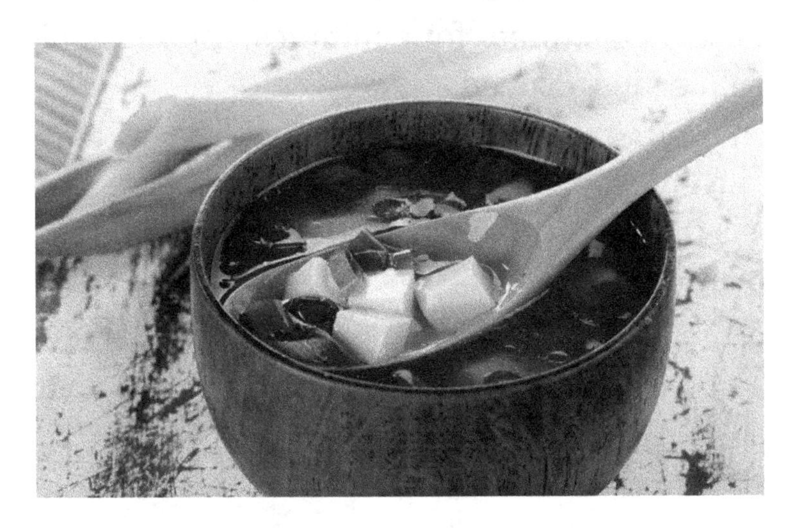

Servings:4
Ingredients:

1 (2-inch) piece wakame
4 cups water
1 medium onion, finely chopped
1 large carrot, finely chopped
2 tbsp. miso, dissolved in 2 tbsp. water
1 tbsp. mirin (sweet rice wine)
1 tbsp. soy sauce
chopped fresh parsley, to garnish

Directions:

Place the wakame in 1 cup of water for 15 minutes; drain. Remove the central rib and cut into small pieces. In a saucepan, boil the remaining water and add the onions, carrots, and wakame pieces. Reduce the heat and simmer for 5 minutes; the vegetables should be just cooked.

Remove from the heat and add the dissolved miso, mirin, and soy sauce. Do not reboil, because this spoils the flavor of the miso. Serve garnished with parsley.

Green Salad & ranch-style Dressing

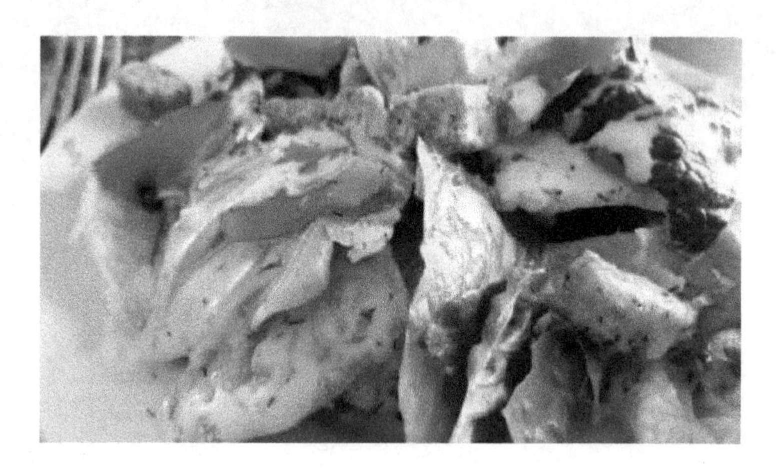

Servings:4
Ingredients:

for the ranch dressing
1/2 cup silken tofu
1/4 cup cider vinegar
2 garlic cloves, minced
2 tbsp. olive oil
1 tsp. Dijon mustard
1 tsp. maple syrup
2 tbsp. minced fresh flat-leaf parsley
1/2 tbsp. fresh oregano
1/4 tbsp. fresh thyme
sea salt and white pepper
oat milk, if required

for the salad

1 head butter lettuce
1 small head radicchio
1 bunch arugula
4 scallions, thinly sliced
1 cup alfalfa sprouts

Directions:

For ranch dressing, put all the ingredients except the salt, pepper, and oat milk in a blender. Process until blended. Taste, season with salt and pepper, and add a little oat milk to thin, if needed. Cover and refrigerate.
To make the salad, wash, dry, and prepare the vegetables, and place in a serving bowl.
Just before serving, pour in enough dressing to lightly coat the salad, toss gently, then serve with additional dressing on the side.

Wheat Berry Salad

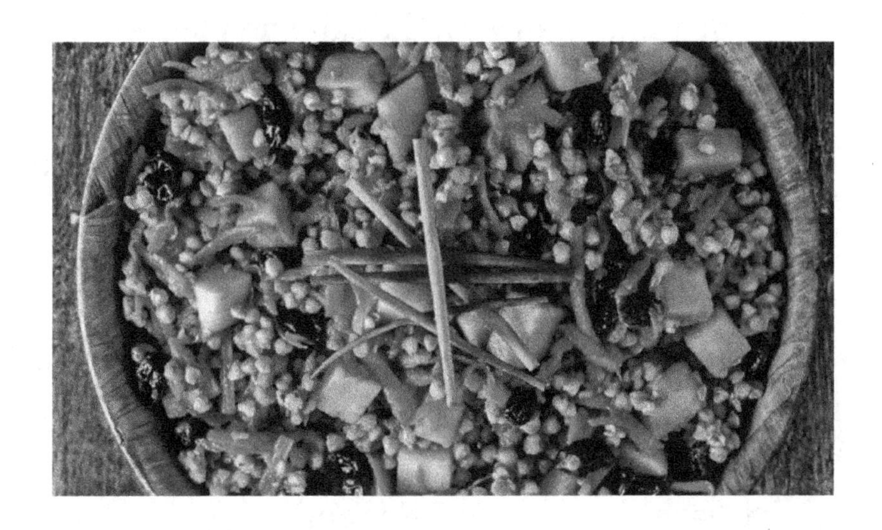

Servings:4
Ingredients:

1 cup wheat berries
1/2 tsp. salt
3 tbsp. olive oil
1 large yellow onion, sliced
1 small red bell pepper, sliced
1 small green bell pepper, sliced
1 small yellow bell pepper, sliced
3 tbsp. tamari soy sauce
2 tbsp. chopped fresh flat-leaf parsley
black pepper
fresh parsley sprigs, to garnish

Directions:

Rinse the wheat berries under cold water, then put them in a saucepan with the salt and plenty of water. Boil and simmer for until tender.
Drain and set aside.
In the meanwhile, heat the olive oil in a large skillet and cook the onion for about 8 minutes, until golden.
Add the sliced peppers and continue to cook until they are soft.
Toss the onions and peppers into the wheat berries with the tamari, chopped parsley, and plenty of black pepper.
Serve garnished with parsley sprigs.

Avocado & Tomato Salad

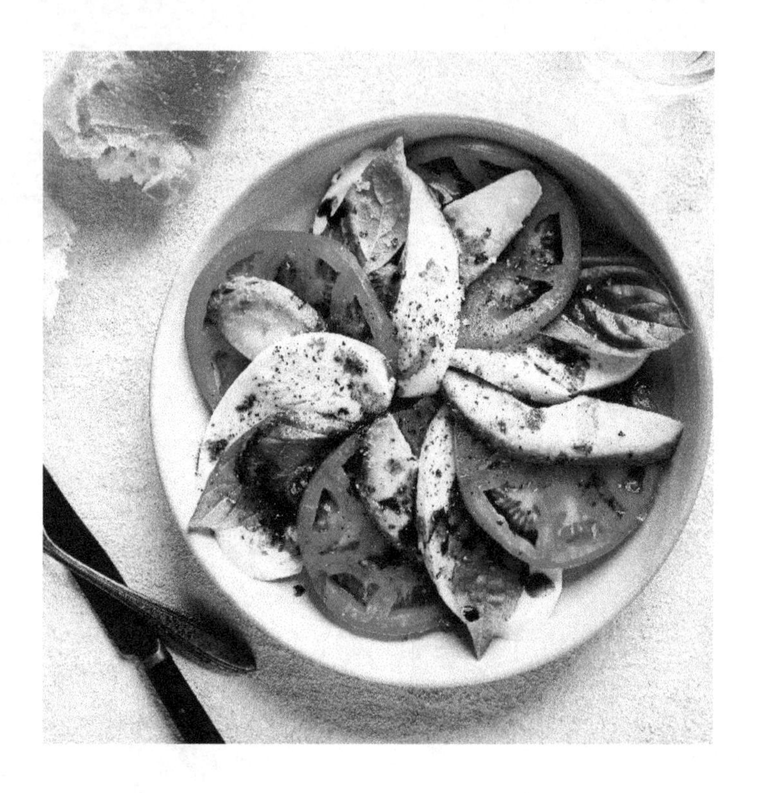

Servings:4
Ingredients:

2 tbsp. pine nuts
2 avocados, peeled, pitted, and sliced
1 tbsp. lemon juice
3 ripe beefsteak tomatoes, roughly chopped
1 small red onion, finely sliced
8 radishes, trimmed and sliced
2 tbsp.fresh basil
salt and black pepper

1 head Romaine lettuce, trimmed and roughly torn
for the dressing
3 tbsp. olive oil
1 tbsp. balsamic vinegar
1 small garlic clove, minced

Directions:

Toast pine nuts in a hot skillet until golden brown, set aside and cool.
Toss the sliced avocado in lemon juice to prevent it browning, then combine with the tomatoes, onions, and radishes. Season with salt and pepper.
Mix together the ingredients for the dressing.
Pour the dressing over the avocado–tomato mixture.
Set aside for at least 20 minutes for the flavors to blend.
Line a salad bowl with the Romaine lettuce, gently add the avocado–tomato mixture, and serve garnished with the pine nuts.

Warm Potato Salad

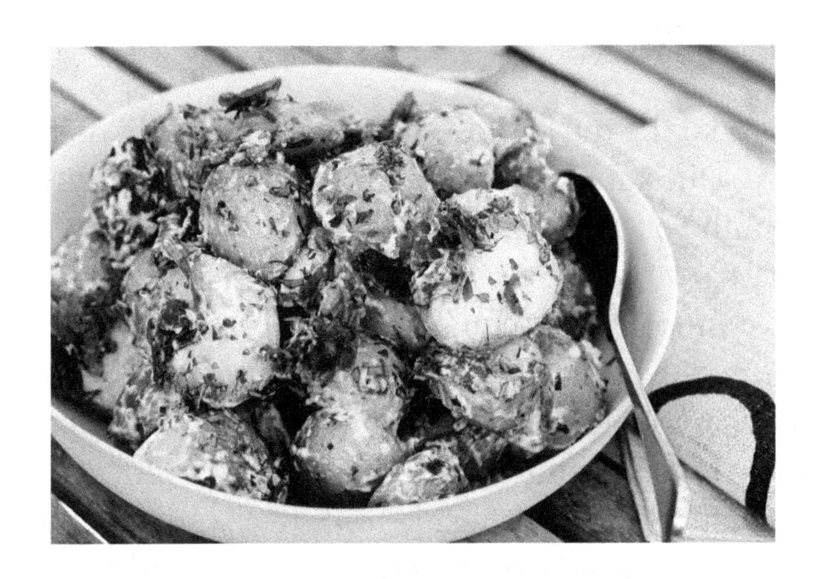

Servings:4
Ingredients:

for the mayonnaise
1/2 cup soy milk
4 tbsp. lemon juice
1/2 tsp. Dijon mustard
pinch paprika
approximately 3/4 cup mixed olive oil and canola oil
sea salt
for the salad
1 1/2 lbs. small red-skinned potatoes, diced
1 tbsp. chopped fresh dill
1 tbsp. snipped fresh chives

1/2 cup finely chopped red onion
sea salt and black pepper

Directions:

To make the mayonnaise, place the soy milk, lemon juice, Dijon mustard, and paprika in a bowl. Whisk to combine or use a blender.
Very slowly add the oil in a gentle stream, whisking constantly, until the mayonnaise is thick, then continue with the mixing for 1 minute longer.
Cook small the potatoes in a pan of boiling salted water for 10 minutes until just tender. Drain and tip into a large bowl. Set aside until just warm. Drizzle the mayonnaise over the potatoes and gently
mix.
Let stand for at least 15 minutes to allow the potatoes to absorb the flavors.
Stir the dill, chives, and red onion into the potatoes, then season to taste with salt and pepper. Serve immediately.

Pear & Endive salad with Caramelized Cashews

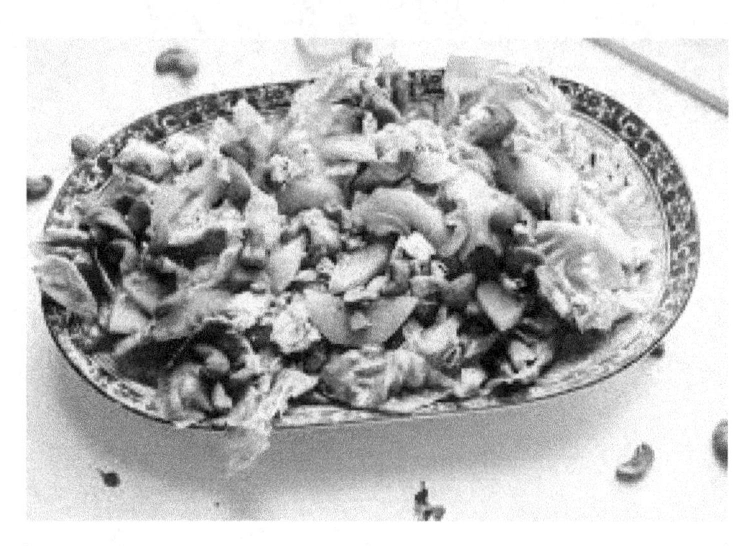

Servings:4
Ingredients:

for the cashews
1/2 cup cashews
2 tsp. vegetable oil
sea salt
1/2 cup maple or agave syrup
for the salad
4 heads Belgian endive
2 ripe pears, unpeeled
for the dressing
2 tbsp. white wine vinegar

1 tsp. Dijon mustard
1 cup olive oil
salt, to taste

Directions:

Line a plate with parchment paper. Preheat a heavy-bottomed pan over a low-medium heat, then toast the cashews for about 5 minutes, tossing them frequently.
Sprinkle the vegetable oil and a little salt over the cashews, and toss to coat. Add the maple or agave syrup, continue to toss for about 30 seconds, until the syrup begins to bubble.
Transfer to the parchment paper and allow to cool completely. Break apart. Separate some large leaves of Belgian endive and arrange them around each individual serving plate in a star pattern.
Chop the remaining endive and place in the center of the dish.
Before serving, combine all the dressing ingredients in a small bowl.
Chop the pears and toss with a little of the salad dressing to prevent the pears from browning, then arrange them over the endive leaves. Sprinkle caramelized cashews over each serving.

Refried Bean Tacos

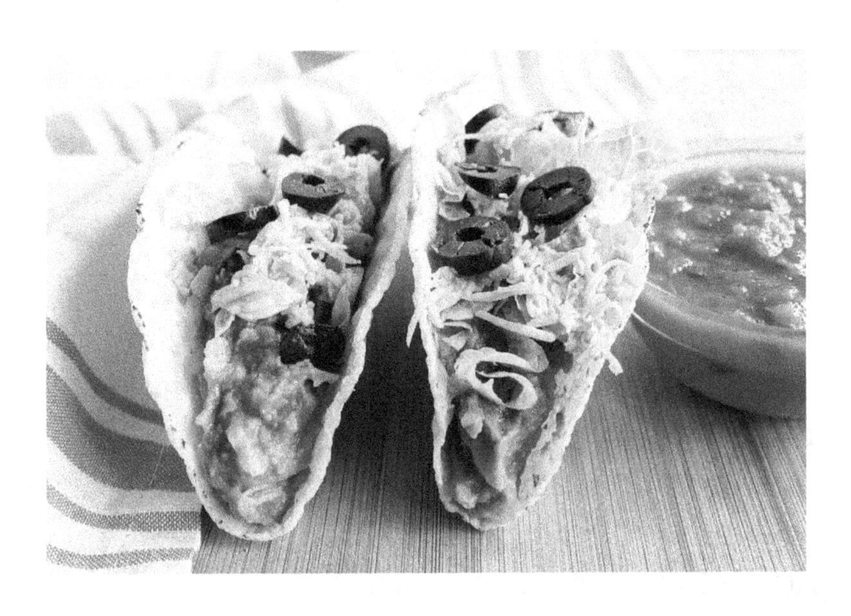

Servings:4
Ingredients:

1 tbsp. sunflower oil
1 small onion, sliced
1 (14-oz.) can vegetarian refried beans
1 (4-oz.) can chopped green chiles, drained
1/4 cup canned crushed tomatoes
1/4 cup black olives, halved
1 cup nondairy "cheese" (cheddar-or Monterey Jack-style)
12 cornmeal taco shells, warmed
for the topping
shredded lettuce

soy yogurt or nondairy sour cream
chopped fresh tomatoes
chopped onion
chopped fresh cilantro

Directions:

Heat the oil in a skillet, add the onion, and cook over a medium-high heat for 5–7 minutes or until the onion is soft. Reduce the heat, then stir in the refried beans, green chiles, tomatoes, and olives. Boiled the mixture, stirring constantly to prevent the beans from scorching.
Stir in the “cheese,” if using.
Put the bean mixture into the warmed taco shells and serve with a selection of the toppings.

Pasta e Fagioli

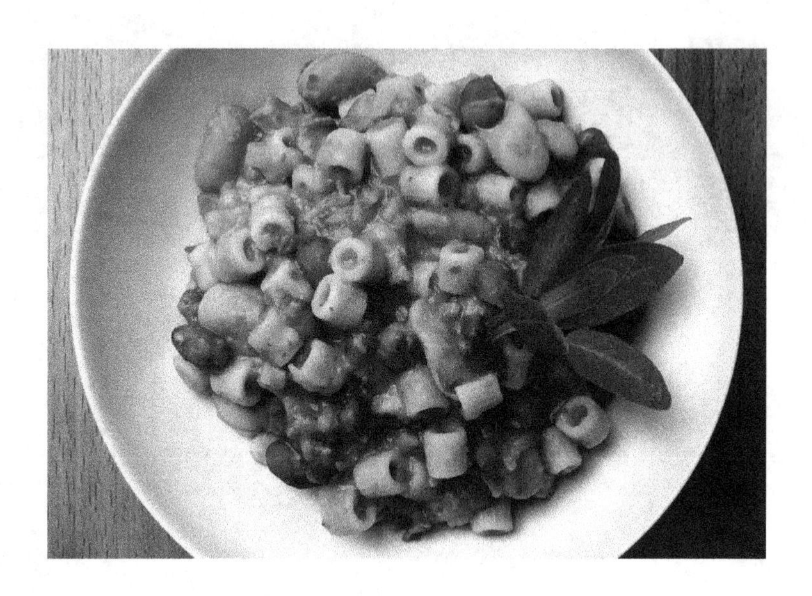

Servings:4
Ingredients:

2 tbsp. olive oil
1 medium onion, finely chopped
1 small carrot, finely chopped
1 stalk celery, finely chopped
4 large cloves garlic, chopped
1 cup canned tomato sauce
1 quart plus 2 cups vegetable bouillon
2 sprigs rosemary, left intact, or 2 tsp. dried rosemary
1 large sprig thyme, left intact, or 1 tsp. dried thyme
1 large fresh bay leaf

1 1/2 cups ditalini or other small pasta
2 (15-oz.) cans cranberry beans
sea salt and black pepper

Directions:

Heat the oil in a large skillet, then add the onion, carrot, and celery.
Cook over medium-high heat for 5–7 minutes or until the onion is soft. Stir in the garlic, tomato sauce or tomatoes, bouillon, and herbs. Boiled then reduce the heat, cover, and simmer for 30 minutes, stirring occasionally.
Return the stew to a rapid boil and add the pasta and beans.
Reduce the heat to low and cook for 10 minutes until the pasta is just cooked.
Remove the herb sprigs, if using, and the bay leaf before serving.

Lentil & Quinoa burgers with Mango Salsa

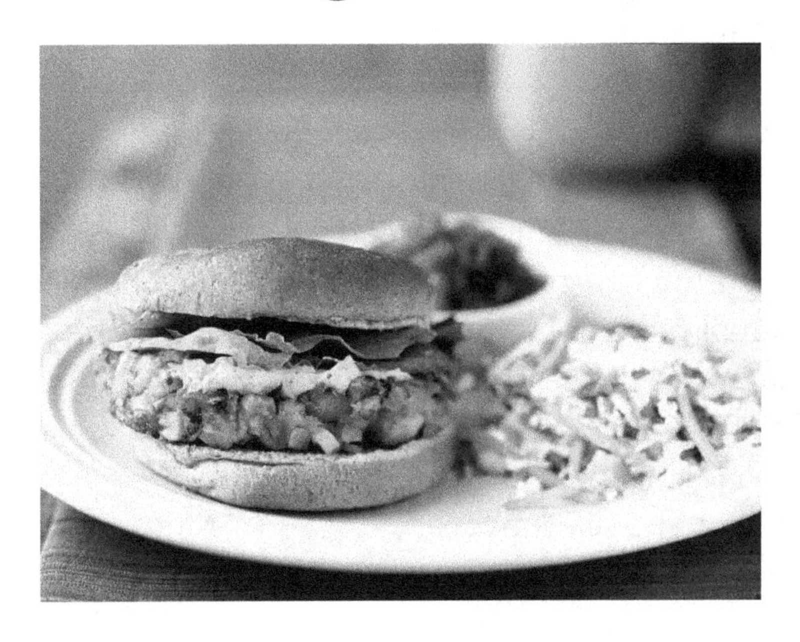

Servings:4
Ingredients:

1 cup green or brown lentils
1/2 cup quinoa
1 tbsp. olive oil
1 small onion, finely chopped
1 small carrot, grated
2 tsp. ground cumin
3/4 cup soft breadcrumbs
2 tbsp. chopped fresh parsley
3 tbsp. tomato paste

1 tbsp. soy sauce
1 tbsp. nutritional yeast
2 tbsp. peanut butter
sea salt and black pepper
cornmeal or oats
for coating
olive oil, for frying
for the mango salsa
1 mango, peeled and chopped
1 medium bell green pepper, seeded and chopped
1 small red onion, finely chopped
1 jalapeño pepper, finely chopped
2 tbsp. lime juice
1 tbsp. pineapple juice or orange juice
sea salt and black pepper
chopped fresh cilantro to garnish

Directions:

Put the lentils and quinoa in a saucepan of boiling water, reduce the heat, and simmer until soft, approximately 20 minutes. Drain and cool, and then use a potato masher to break down the lentils.

To make the salsa, combine all the ingredients in a bowl and set aside.

Meanwhile, heat the oil in a medium skillet, add the onion, and cook over a medium-high heat for 5–7 minutes or until it is soft. Stir in the carrots

and cumin, and cook for 2 minutes.
Combine the lentil-quinoa mixture with onions and carrots. Stir in the breadcrumbs, parsley, tomato paste, soy sauce, nutritional yeast, and peanut butter. Knead the mixture with your hands until combined. Form the mixture into 8 burgers.
Coat each burger in a little cornmeal or oats. Chill, if desired, until ready to cook.
To serve, heat 1 tablespoon olive oil in a skillet and fry the burgers over medium-low heat until crisp and golden on each side, 4–5 minutes. Serve with the mango salsa.

Tomato Farinata

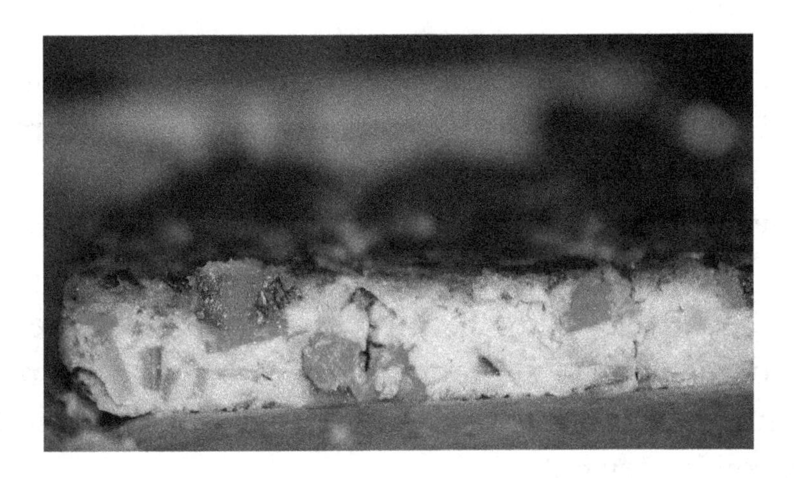

Servings:4
Ingredients:

for the farinata
1 cup gram (garbanzo) flour
1 tsp. sea salt
1 cup plus 2 tbsp. warm water
4 tbsp. olive oil
black pepper
for the topping
2 ripe tomatoes, skinned, seeded, and chopped
2 scallions, sliced
4 black olives, quartered
1/2 tsp. red pepper flakes (optional)
1 tbsp. chopped fresh rosemary
1 tsp. lemon juice

sea salt and black pepper

Directions:

Sift in the gram flour in a plastic bowl and add the salt. Pour in the water, constantly stirring, to form a thin, smooth batter.
Cover for 2 hours with a damp tea towel and let rest in a warm place.
Preheat oven to 425°F. Stir 3 tablespoons of olive oil into the batter. Put the remaining oil in an 8×8-inch baking pan, then put the pan in the oven briefly until the oil is very hot.
Pour in the batter, and arrange the topping ingredients on the surface, sprinkling the surface evenly with each in turn. Bake for about 15 minutes, until golden and crisp. Serve hot or at room temperature.

DESSERT

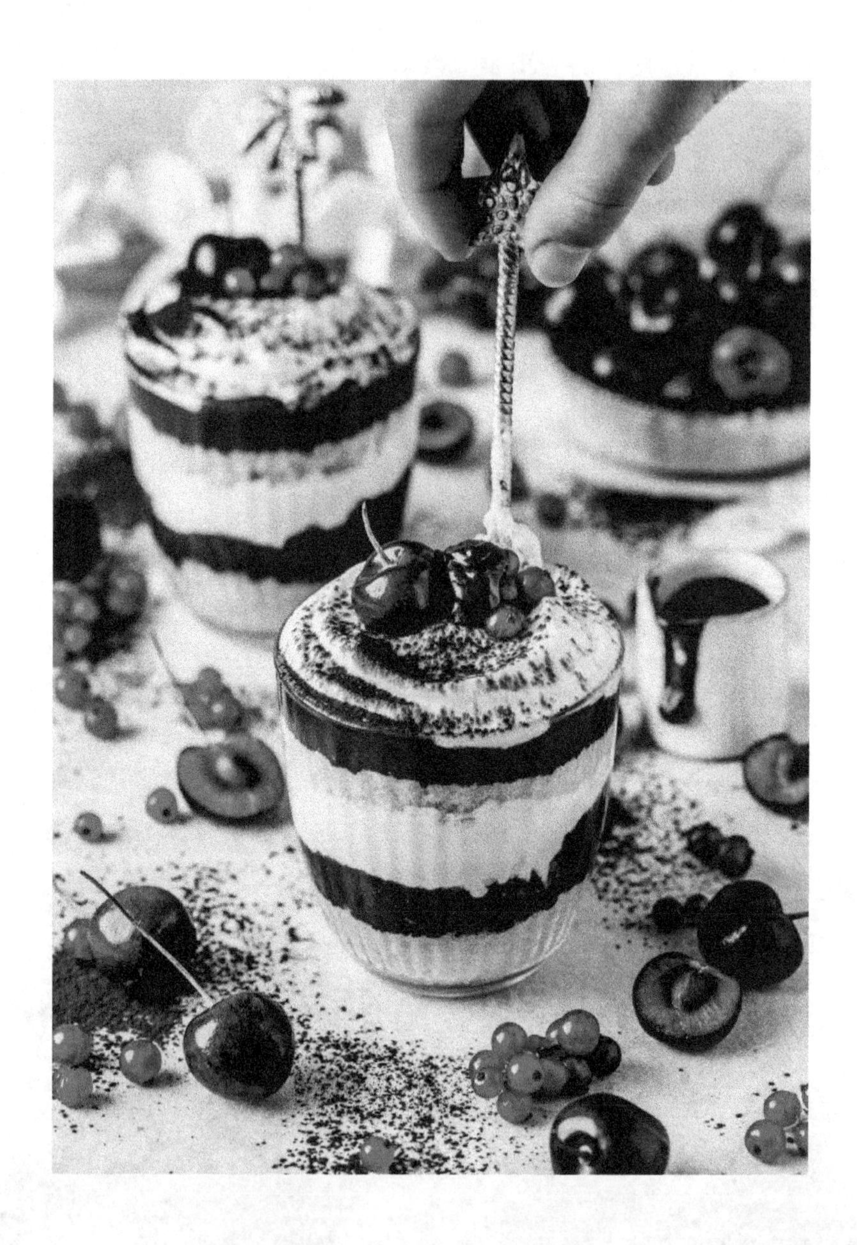

Silken Chocolate Mousse

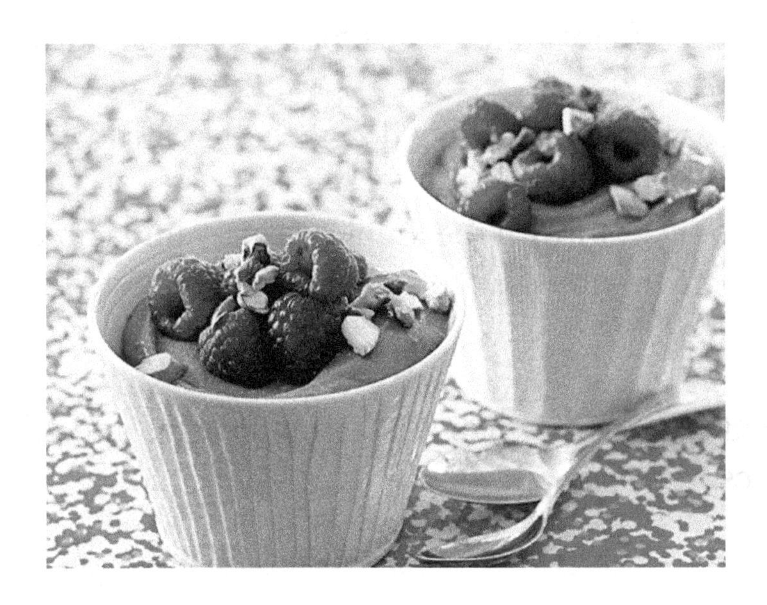

Servings:4
Ingredients:

1 (12-oz.) package silken tofu, room temperature, drained
10 oz. semisweet vegan chocolate
3 tbsp. maple syrup
1 tsp. vanilla extract
2 tbsp. amaretto or a few drops almond extract
fresh raspberries and mint leaves, to garnish

Directions:

Beat the tofu by hand or in a food processor until smooth.

Melt vegan chocolate in a double boiler, stirring frequently until smooth.

Add to the tofu with the maple syrup, vanilla, and amaretto or almond extract, and beat by hand to combine.

Pour into small dishes and chill for at least 30 minutes. Serve garnished with raspberries and mint leaves.

Apple Strudel

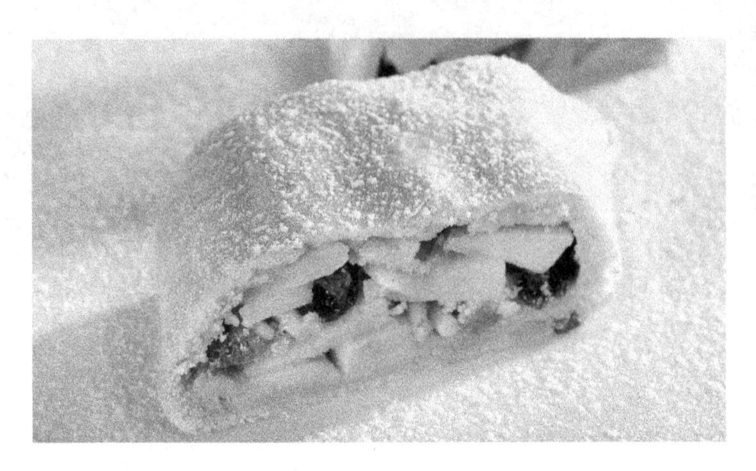

Servings:4
Ingredients:

zest and juice of 1/2 lemon
4 medium Granny Smith apples
1/2 cup finely chopped pecans
1/2 cup soft, fresh breadcrumbs
2 tsp. ground cinnamon
3/4 cup brown sugar
4–6 sheets phyllo pastry (12×17-inch)
1/4 cup canola oil
1/2 cup golden raisins
confectioners' sugar, to finish

Directions:

Preheat the oven to 350°F. Fill a bowl with cold water and add the lemon juice. Peel and slice the apples, dropping the slices into the water to prevent them from browning. In a separate bowl, combine the pecans, breadcrumbs, cinnamon, and 1/2 cup of brown sugar.

Put the first sheet of phyllo pastry on a clean kitchen towel on your work surface and
brush with oil. Sprinkle with a third of the pecan mixture.

Put another sheet of phyllo pastry on top, brush with oil, and sprinkle with another third of the pecan mixture; repeat with the third sheet, then lay the fourth sheet on top.

Drain the apples and pat dry, then mix them with the remaining sugar, lemon zest, and golden raisins. Lay the apples evenly along the length of the phyllo but no more than halfway across it and leaving a 1/2-inch margin around the edges.

Brush the edges with a little water. Roll up the dough lengthwise, like a jelly roll, using the cloth to help support the dough; press your strudel together gently.

Place the strudel on a silicone sheet or on parchment paper on a cookie sheet, and bake until golden brown(25 min.).

Serve hot or at room temperature. Serve sprinkled with confectioners' sugar, with a scoop of non-dairy ice cream. If you wish, the strudel may be made ahead of time and reheated for 10 minutes in a hot oven.

Baked Rice Pudding

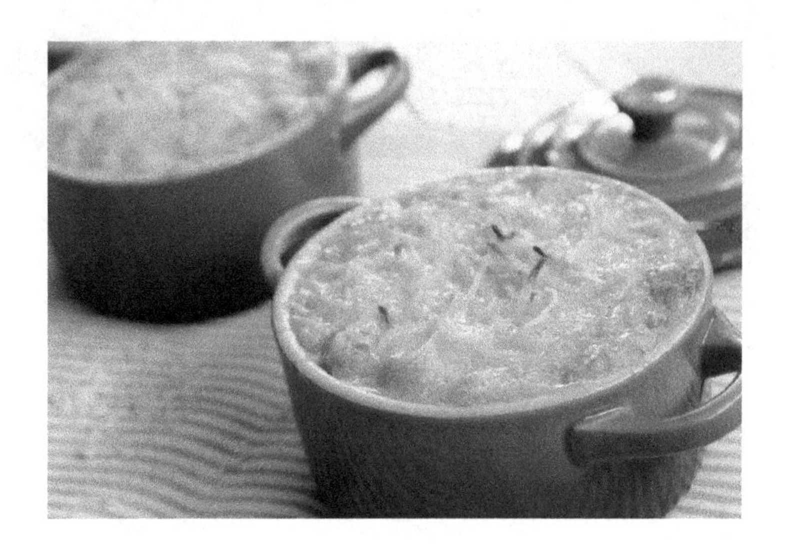

Servings:4
Ingredients:

5 tbsp. short-grain rice
3 tbsp. Brown sugar or 2 tbsp. agave syrup
1 strip lemon zest or 1 vanilla pod
4 1/2 cups soy or other unsweetened nondairy milk
1/4 tsp. grated nutmeg
2 tbsp. nondairy margarine or butter

Directions:

Preheat oven to 300°F. Generously grease a 1-quart ovenproof dish with non-dairy butter or margarine. Put the rice, brown sugar or syrup, and lemon zest or vanilla pod in the dish. Gently pour in the milk and stir.

Sprinkle the grated nutmeg over the surface of the milk and dot with butter or margarine.

Carefully transfer to the oven and bake for 40 minutes, stir, then let cook for another 75 minutes, by which time a brown crust will have formed and the rice will be fully cooked. Serve hot.

Tropical Fruit Kebabs

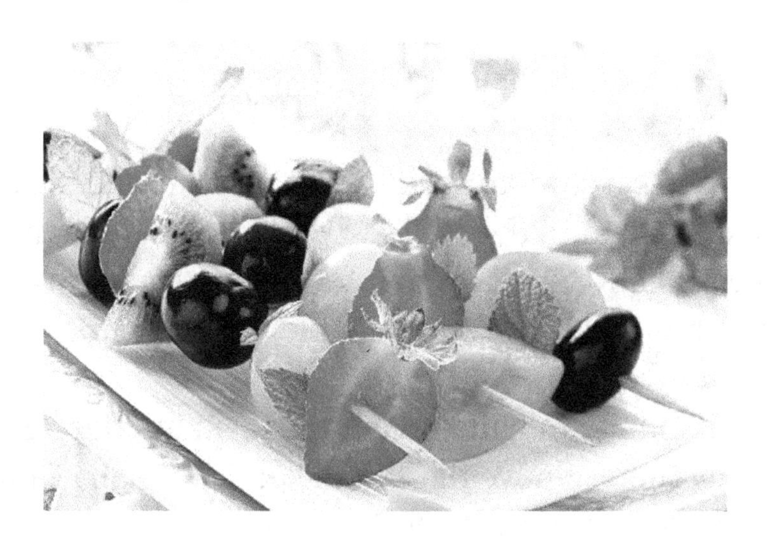

Servings:4
Ingredients:

for the syrup
1/3 cup non-dairy butter
1/3 cup maple syrup
6 cardamom pods, seeds only
1 whole clove
1 (3-inch) cinnamon stick
1/2 tsp. vanilla extract
for the kebabs
1/2 small pineapple
2 ripe mangoes
2 firm bananas
non-dairy ice cream serve

Directions:

In a large skillet, melt the non-dairy butter and stir in the maple syrup.
Crush the cardamom seeds with a mortar and pestle, then add them to the syrup with the clove, cinnamon, and vanilla. Keep warm to infuse while preparing the fruit. Skin and core the pineapple and cut into 1-inch chunks.
Cut the mango in half and cut the flesh into large chunks, then remove the skin. Peel the bananas and cut into 1-inch slices.
Thread the fruit onto 8 metal skewers or wooden skewers that have been soaked in water for 30 minutes to prevent burning. Preheat the barbecue coals or the broiler to medium-hot. Remove the clove and cinnamon stick from the syrup.
Put the kebabs on an oiled rack and cook, turning once, and frequently basting with the syrup until the fruit is lightly browned on the outside, about 5 minutes. Do not overcook or the fruit will fall apart.
Drizzle with any remaining syrup and serve immediately with non-dairy ice cream or non-dairy yogurt.

Soy Chocolate Ice Cream

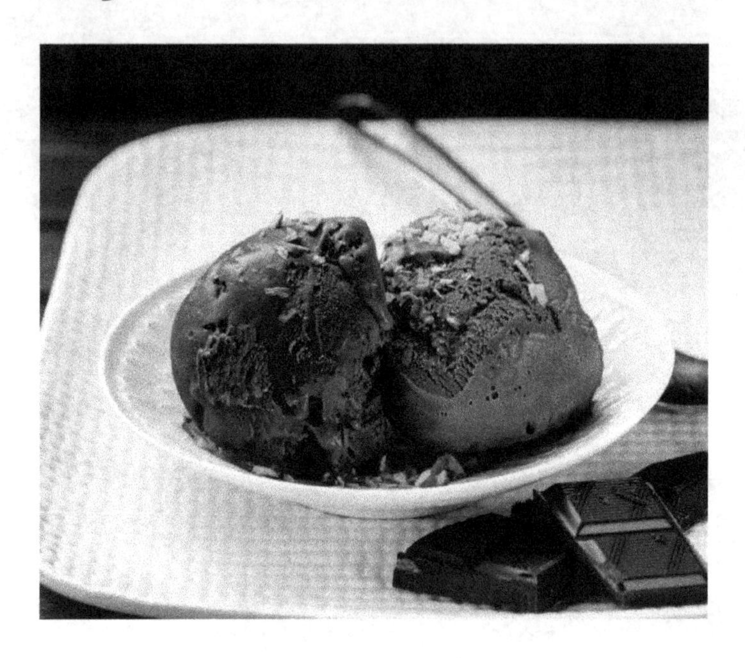

Servings:4
Ingredients:

2 tbsp. arrowroot
1 cup soy milk
2 cups nondairy cream
1/4 cup agave syrup or 1/3 cup sugar
2 tsp. vanilla extract
1 cup small chips of semisweet vegan chocolate
for the chocolate sauce
1/4 cup (1/2 stick) nondairy butter
3/4 cup brown sugar

2 oz. semisweet vegan chocolate, chopped
3–4 tbsp. soy milk

Directions:

Mix the arrowroot to a paste with 2 tablespoons of the soy milk; set aside. In a saucepan, combine the remaining milk, nondairy cream, and syrup or sugar, and bring to a boil.
While stirring, pour the arrowroot paste into the pan, stirring until the mixture thickens slightly.
As it cools the mixture will continue to thicken then cover the surface with greased parchment paper to prevent a skin from forming.
When the mixture is cool, stir in the vanilla extract and the chocolate chips.
Pour the mixture into an ice cream maker and process until the ice cream has set. Alternatively, place in a freezer container and freeze for about 6 hours. Remove from the freezer every 1 1/2 hours and mash with a fork to break down the ice crystals to form a smooth ice cream.
To make the sauce, melt the nondairy butter or margarine in a pan, add the sugar,stirring, over low heat until melted. Add the chocolate and 3 tablespoons soy milk, stir until melted, and add a little more soy milk, if desired. Serve hot over the ice cream.

Toffee Bananas With Coconut Cream

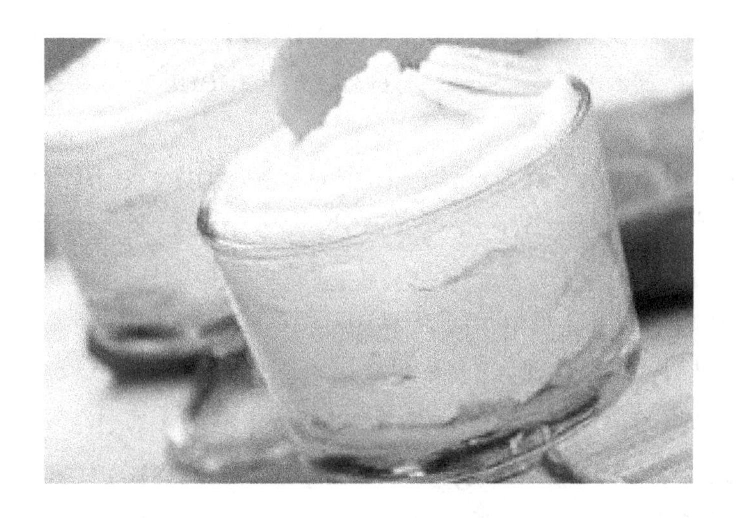

Servings:4
Ingredients:

for the coconut cream
4 oz. block creamed coconut
1/3 cup coconut milk
1/4 cup soy yogurt
4 firm, ripe bananas
1 tbsp. lemon juice
2 tbsp. brown sugar
pinch ground cinnamon
pinch ground nutmeg
toasted coconut, to garnish

Directions:

To make the coconut cream, roughly chop the block of creamed coconut into pieces, and put them in a saucepan with the coconut milk. Heat slowly until the coconut has melted, stirring frequently. Remove and let cool.

Add the yogurt to the cooled coconut cream, beating until the mixture resembles whipped cream in texture.

Let cool and keep refrigerated until required.

Peel the bananas, cut them in half lengthwise, brush with lemon juice, and put in a shallow pan. Sprinkle with the brown sugar and a pinch of cinnamon and nutmeg.

Put under a medium-hot broiler until the sugar is beginning to caramelize and the bananas are soft.

Serve hot with the coconut cream and garnish with toasted coconut.

Strawberry Tart

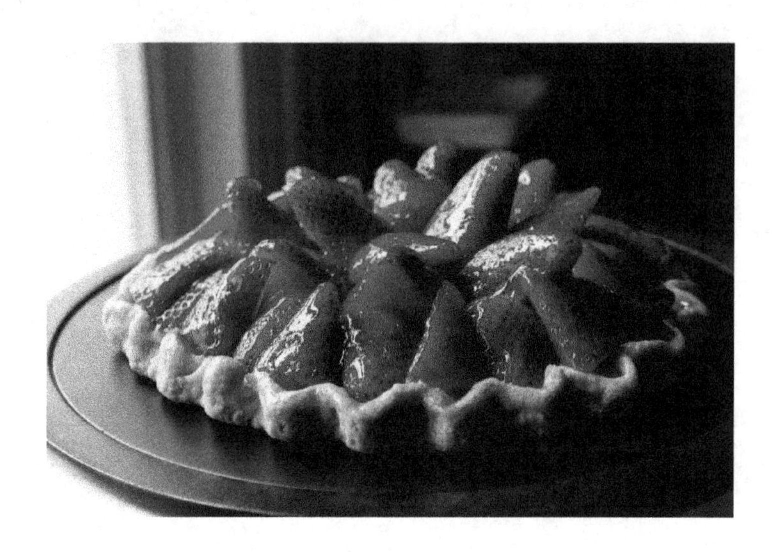

Servings:4
Ingredients:

1 recipe whole wheat pie crust (see recipe)
1 lb. ripe strawberries, halved
small fresh mint leaves
for the glaze
1/2 cup sugar
1/4 cup cornstarch
1 cup water
1/4 cup strawberry preserves
1 tbsp. lemon juice

Directions:

Preheat oven to 400°F. Lightly butter a 9-inch tart pan. Roll out the pie crust on a floured surface, use it to line the tart pan, and chill for 20 minutes. Line the base of the pie crust with parchment weighted down with pie weights or baking beans, then bake for 12 minutes.
Reduce the heat to 230°F and bake for 10 minutes more. Remove the parchment and beans and cook for another 10 minutes for the crust to dry out. Cool.
To make the glaze, mix together all the glaze ingredients in a saucepan.
Bring to a boil stirring for few minute, until thickened.
Remove from heat and cool slightly.
Spread half of the warm glaze over the cooked crust.
Top with the strawberries, then brush the remaining warm glaze over the strawberries. Let cool and serve cold, garnished with small mint leaves.

Conclusions

I am sure that the recipes I have written in this book have helped you to increase your culinary skills on Vegan cooking and if you are a beginner it has definitely given you an important base to create your own dishes as well...

Thank you for choosing my book and I look forward to seeing you in the next cookbook.

Create, Cook and Live Healthy.

CPSIA information can be obtained
at www.ICGtesting.com
Printed in the USA
BVHW091136270521
608294BV00002B/281

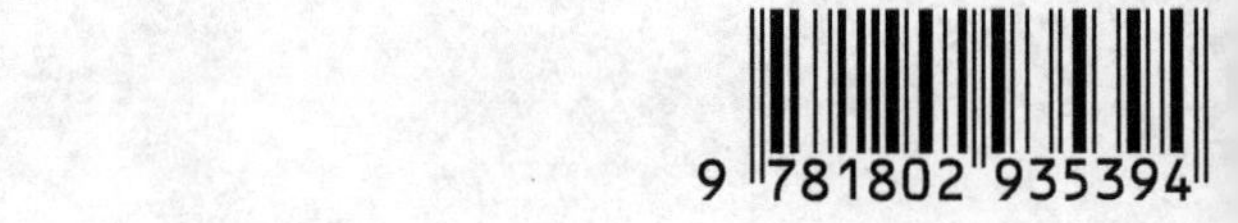